In Praise
The Health Care Consumer's Manifesto

"Deb Gordon takes a fresh look at health care spending in the U.S. She breaks through the mystery of health care and shows how people can thrive in the health system."

—David Cutler,
Otto Eckstein Professor of Applied Economics, Harvard University

"Like a trusted friend who knows exactly what she's talking about, Deb Gordon guides us masterfully through the health care maze . . . encouraging and empowering consumers to navigate their own unique challenges. There is hope! We need this book more than ever."

—Jane Clayson Johnson, former ABC and CBS news
correspondent and cohost of CBS's *The Early Show*;
author, *Silent Souls Weeping*

"As a patient and a medical provider, I am grateful for this book. It is packed with wisdom and practical advice with the power to improve the health care experience, and ultimately health outcomes, for all. Through personal stories, it captures the essence of what is broken in health care today—a system built on the flawed assumption that the doctor always knows best—and reminds us that we all have the ability and the right to speak out and be heard."

—Annie Brewster, MD,
founder and executive director, Health Story Collaborative;
assistant professor, Harvard Medical School;
associate physician, Massachusetts General Hospital

"We are in a consumer-driven economy. Many of us spend more time thinking about our next cup of coffee than we do our own health care. *The Health Care Consumer's Manifesto* takes a close look at health care today and shines a light on how consumers can and should be more active and informed about their well-being."

—Paul Matsen,
chief marketing and communications officer, Cleveland Clinic

"Finally, a guide to health care written entirely with the consumer's priorities in mind. Deborah Dove Gordon has given us a richly informative, ultra-practical guide with a wealth of useful information from how to get price transparency on health care procedures to how we can use our consumer power to change the system as a whole. Empowering, honest, and refreshingly straight forward, this is one of those books that will likely pay for itself hundreds of times over in avoided costs."

—Shannon Coulter, president, Grab Your Wallet Alliance

"Deb Gordon does away with tired old arguments against price transparency and goes right to the heart of the matter: where else would consumers be expected to pay without first knowing the price? This book shines a bright spotlight on the secrecy and confusion around health care pricing, and shows consumers how they can get to the price information they need to make informed health care choices."

—Barbara Anthony, Senior Fellow in Healthcare,
Pioneer Institute and former Massachusetts
Undersecretary of the Office of Consumer
Affairs and Business Regulation

"At a critical time in the transformation of the American health care system, Deb Gordon provides a terrific libretto for this most complex and incomprehensible opera. She brilliantly empowers American consumers to better access and demand real value and quality for what are truly the most important services and products that they can access for their families and themselves."

—Gary L. Gottlieb, MD, MBA,
professor of psychiatry, Harvard Medical School;
former president and CEO, Partners Healthcare System;
former CEO, Partners in Health

"For markets to function properly, consumers need access to information about prices and quality as well as meaningful choice. This 'Manifesto' doesn't just document how badly these conditions fail in health care; it explains why our current system won't deliver better outcomes unless health care consumers become a force for change."

—Susan Athey,
economics of technology professor,
Stanford University Graduate School of Business

"In *The Health Care Consumer's Manifesto*, Deborah Gordon explores in depth the fact that despite spending over a trillion dollars and rising out of pocket on health care, we rarely use our power as consumers to get the best quality and lower price. She explores why this is currently so, why this is changing, and what consumers can do to hasten this change. A must read for anyone who has been frustrated with the experience, quality, or cost of health care in the U.S.; and for providers, payers, and policy makers to prepare for the new world to come."

—Rushika Fernandopulle, MD, MPP, CEO, Iora Health

"Deb Gordon has captured the pain of dealing with health care and how it can be worse than the pain of illness itself for consumers. Until we align the interests of patients, payers, and providers in new models of payment and care delivery, we will continue to see consumers challenged by the illogical and unkind structures of a system built for a different time. New market entrants recognize the importance of consumer experience and trust; traditional health care entities must begin to think of consumers as customers who are paying for a third of health care expenditures or more. The book brings readers deep into consumer mind-sets, revealing the depth to which consumers are struggling with their evolving role as health care buyers. Anyone trying to understand what it means to be engaged in the American health care system, especially as a consumer, should read this book and think hard about how to rebuild a system that is meant to treat the hearts and minds of consumers, but has lost touch with those organs along the way."

—Lisa Suennen, venture capital investor, industry advisor,
entrepreneur, and leading voice in digital health;
author, Venture Valkyrie blog; cohost, Tech Tonics podcast;
cofounder, CSweetener; Rock Health Top
Digital Health Evangelist (2018);
University of California Berkeley Haas faculty member

"This is an important book that serves as a call to action from every health care consumer, because it addresses the most critical issue with our health care system, cost of care and how empowered patients must begin to take charge of their personal experiences with the system. Full of poignant anecdotal stories, *The Health Care Consumer's Manifesto* includes excellent guidelines on how to determine and negotiate the cost of a procedure or treatment; how to understand the parameters of various insurance programs; and most importantly how to assert your voice as an activated e-patient. For every individual who is frustrated with the system and grappling with how to manage their cost of care, this is a must read."

—Nancy B. Finn, health care journalist, author of
*e-Patients Live Longer: The Complete Guide to
Managing Health Care Using Technology* and
Digital Communication in Medical Practice

"A sassy, upbeat manifesto for how Americans should get more from health care."

—Camilla Cavendish, author,
Extra Time: Ten Lessons for an Aging World

The Health Care
Consumer's Manifesto

The Health Care Consumer's Manifesto

HOW TO GET THE MOST FOR YOUR MONEY

Deborah Dove Gordon

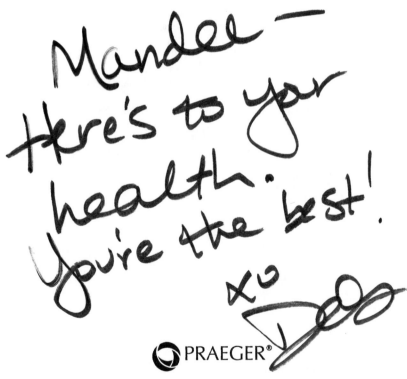

Mandee —
Here's to your
health.
You're the best!
xo
Deb

PRAEGER®

An Imprint of ABC-CLIO, LLC

Santa Barbara, California • Denver, Colorado

Library of Congress Cataloging-in-Publication Data

Names: Gordon, Deborah D. (Deborah Dove), author.
Title: The health care consumer's manifesto : how to get the most for your money /
    Deborah Dove Gordon.
Description: Santa Barbara, California : Praeger, an imprint of ABC-CLIO, LLC,
    [2020] | Includes bibliographical references and index.
Identifiers: LCCN 2019051171 (print) | LCCN 2019051172 (ebook) |
    ISBN 9781440874048 (hardcover: alk. paper) | ISBN 9781440874055 (ebook)
Subjects: LCSH: Medical care, Cost of—United States. | Medical care—
    United States. | Consumer education—United States. | Patient education—
    United States.
Classification: LCC RA410.53 .G67 2020 (print) | LCC RA410.53 (ebook) |
    DDC 338.4/3362104258—dc23
LC record available at https://lccn.loc.gov/2019051171
LC ebook record available at https://lccn.loc.gov/2019051172

ISBN: 978-1-4408-7404-8 (print)
    978-1-4408-7755-1 (paperback)
    978-1-4408-7405-5 (ebook)

24 23 22 21 20   1 2 3 4 5

This book is also available as an eBook.

Praeger
An Imprint of ABC-CLIO, LLC

ABC-CLIO, LLC
147 Castilian Drive
Santa Barbara, California 93117
www.abc-clio.com

This book is printed on acid-free paper ∞

Manufactured in the United States of America

To consumers everywhere—with vast hope for what we can do together to transform health care.

And to Roy, Zoë, Jasper, and Tiny—with infinite love and gratitude.

Contents

Part Two: The Consumer Manifesto

Part Three: Getting Better

Acknowledgments

I am grateful for the support that enabled this project, including from my agent Sara Camilli and the team at Praeger.

Without the consumers who trusted me with their stories, this book would not exist.

Thanks to the many friends who said "You should!" when I wondered aloud about writing a book and specifically to Kate Novack, Lexie Olmsted, Lauren Sandler, and Dolma Tsering for their help. Every first-time author should be so lucky to have writer friends like Emily Franklin and Michelle Icard, who each generously offered me tangible advice and moral support throughout this process.

At Provincetown's Fine Arts Work Center, Lacy M. Johnson and Sarah Green helped me conceptualize and start this book. The Provincetown Commons and countless cafés provided white-noise havens in which to finish it.

Thanks to Professors John Haigh, Joseph Newhouse, and Richard Zeckhauser for giving me a home base at the Harvard Kennedy School and to the senior fellows for friendship and camaraderie. Special thanks to Scott Leland and Susan Gill for their support; John Della Volpe for the RealClear Politics collaboration; and my outstanding research assistants Joemma Berberich, Julie-Ann Hutchinson, Akshaya Kannan, Gwendolyn Lee, Ihsaan Patel, Amelia Pellegrini, William Tran, Natalie Triedman, and especially Anna Ford—my thought partner throughout. Thanks, too, to Dana Ellis, Catherine Leslie, and the MIT AgeLab.

Thanks to my parents Alice and Martin Gordon, who taught me to use my voice unapologetically; my sister Anne Gordon for exquisite editing; and my extended family for their love and input.

Endless thanks to Zoë and Jasper for tolerating this process and for letting me peek at the world through their astute and compassionate lenses;

Tiny for ferociously guarding me; and most of all Roy, for convincing me I could do this and should, for keeping us all fed, for reading everything from the roughest kernels to final-final drafts, and for the best advice I got: "Just write!"

NOTE

Throughout this book, I share stories of real consumers. I refer to them by aliases to protect their anonymity. Because most consumer interviews were recorded and transcribed, the quotes are largely verbatim, edited only for length and clarity.

PART ONE

Consumer Power

Introduction: A Nation of Shoppers

Shopping our way to a better health care system

Americans love to shop. We shop for gadgets, airline tickets, new outfits, the latest smartphone. We even shop for things we may not love, like mortgages and home repairs. We love the act of shopping almost as much as the goods themselves, especially in the digital age. The Internet lets us shop from home, on the road, at the coffee shop. We share stories about our purchases in real time. Americans expect to get what we pay for and often feel empowered to demand accountability for our purchase experiences. If Amazon screws up an order, we expect them to fix it, and they invariably do. If a restaurant mixes up our order, many of us will eat it anyway, but some of us will send it back and get the food we wanted. We catalogue our meals and indulgences, capturing and publishing our every consumer experience. We tweet angrily to stores or airlines or banks that wrong us, give us bad service, and don't listen or respond to our needs. Social media gives us newfound power, which we use to publicly shame powerful corporations to extract a sort of vigilante consumer justice.

But at the doctor's office, in the hospital, or in a dentist's chair, we tend not to stand up for ourselves the same way. We don't shop around for a better price on a service we are told we need and don't question. We usually don't know—or even think to ask—what the price will be in the first place. We seek shortcuts to protect ourselves from the soul-sucking process of choosing health insurance, uncomfortable imagining our future risks and unable to calculate their projected costs.

A New York City–based filmmaker told me how she broke up with her longtime therapist like a 7th grader might end her first romance. After years watching her therapist's obvious cognitive decline, sometimes forgetting they had set an appointment or falling asleep mid-session, she simply stopped making appointments and avoided his calls when he checked up on her. Another consumer, the mother of three adult children, didn't storm out in disgust when her dentist failed to wash his hands before examining her. It wasn't until the next visit or the one after that that she finally spoke up and then chose not to return. Inertia, fear, confusion, and respect—however misplaced—are powerful forces.

Would we return to a restaurant whose waiters repeatedly forgot we were there, hungrily awaiting attention? Or to one where we knew the kitchen staff did not follow the bathroom edict that employees must wash their hands before returning to work? Why, then, don't we use our voice, and vote with our feet and our wallets, in health care?

Why do we pay so much for health care in America and get so little? And why, as we are on the hook for more of the health care tab, do Americans tolerate a system that does not serve us better? What might happen if we expected, and then demanded, more value for our health care dollars—like we do when we buy virtually anything else?

I remember hearing a story on National Public Radio (NPR) about a girl whose family had fallen on hard times. I was probably around 8 or 10 years old, and I think the girl in the interview was a little older than I was, maybe 12 or 14. Aware of her family's financial hardship, she talked about taking just half a plate of food at dinner, telling her mother she wasn't hungry but actually trying to help stretch their meal across the family. Should *I* eat less? I remember wondering. Were my parents going without so I could have as much food as I wanted?

My parents' business had taken a downturn. I didn't understand the details, but where their consulting company had once occupied an entire building—whose darkened halls I would roam endlessly on weekends while my parents worked—they had moved into a suite in a building across the street, once their overflow space and now the entire operation. I vaguely understood it to be Ronald Reagan's fault. My parents' government contract work dried up, and so too did my blind comfort in our material status.

During this period, the migraines I had always suffered sporadically—usually in response to an éclair or other dairy-laden food—started appearing almost every day, inexplicably. Worried, my mother took me to a neurologist for a consultation. We didn't have health insurance and frequented an urgent-care, walk-in clinic, paying the flat fee if we were sick.

My mom now says it wasn't a big concern to go without health insurance at that time; medical costs were lower overall, and insurance was designed more explicitly for catastrophic events. There was less stigma of not having health insurance. Our pay-as-you-go approach seemed to work. It seemed accessible and open when we needed it. But I recall sensing this wasn't how most people got their health care, though I didn't understand why. My mom had a knack for being ahead of her time.

Frequent headaches weren't on par with something like a strep test, and I gathered they could signal something pretty bad to warrant a trip to a specialist. "Does your head hurt on one side?" the neurologist asked. Yes. "Does the pain feel like it's pressing in or pushing out?" I had no idea. After a few more questions and some basic tests, the doctor declared, "It does seem that you have migraines."

I cringed watching my mother write a check for an expert to conclude what we had known for years. I didn't think that check, probably for a few hundred dollars, was easy to write. As an adult, I can now see that ruling out something much worse was probably well worth the peace of mind it gave my parents. At the time, though, I could only wish I had never reported the headaches and avoided what seemed like a complete waste of money I didn't think we had.

For my family then, health care was a commodity we'd buy as we needed it. Here, we'd paid for something but gotten what I perceived to be of little value in return. It was as if we'd gone to a restaurant that never served the meal but still brought the check. Worse, at this restaurant, it was taboo to negotiate or stand up for yourself, demanding the food for which you'd been charged.

"Can I come over?" my friend Dara cried over the phone. "We got a letter saying we won't have health insurance starting Friday. I don't know what to do."

Within the hour, Dara arrived, clutching the distressing mail. In the 10 years we had known her, she had gotten married, had her own child, and was saving money to buy a house. She had gotten her U.S. citizenship just the summer before.

The letter had arrived from her husband's employer dated May 10 informing them that the company would no longer carry the family on the company's health insurance plan, effective May 14. Dara's husband, Kiri, had not been at work for many months. His stomach cancer had gone undiagnosed for nearly a year despite several doctor visits. Stomach pain in a young, healthy person must be muscular. No? Well, try antacids. And on it went, until a nurse took a closer look.

Because he was only 35, fit and strong, and because Dara was in denial of the data showing that almost no one survives his type of cancer, they chose to have most of the offending stomach removed altogether. The surgeon called the procedure a Hail Mary, but Dara heard only the next step in his fight. Of course, he would take it. He had to live.

Now, after months of bouncing in and out of the hospital with fevers whose source the doctors could not find, he had been admitted to one of the most expensive hospitals in the country, and the family was about to be without health insurance coverage.

"Are you a lawyer?" the HR manager asked when I called the employer to ask for an explanation. "I'm a family friend," I explained. "I am just curious how you decided to drop them now? What is the policy?" The woman awkwardly told me they try to figure out if the employee is likely to come back to work. She did not say, "We assume he's going to die. He's no longer of use to us." They had no written policy for this.

"Do you think he'll be coming back to work?" she asked, in case they'd assessed his chances incorrectly. This company had already done more than was required by law. They had generously allowed the family to stay on the company health plan during Kiri's long-term leave. Now the company was making an economically rational decision that he was, effectively, no longer an employee—no longer their responsibility. "He's fighting for his life right now," I couldn't resist laying on guilt it seemed she knew she deserved. "He is certainly in no condition to work." It didn't change their decision.

The health insurance part of the story ended well. Having worked for a health plan, I had ideas on where to begin and whom to call for help. When I asked questions—unencumbered by fear of personal financial ruin and a partner-less life—I had a context in which to understand the answers. More important than speaking English, which Dara also does perfectly well, I spoke the inscrutable insider jargon of insurance. The family qualified for publicly sponsored health insurance in a state that wants people to be covered. They wound up paying less than they had on the employer plan and faced no gap in coverage. When Kiri died in that hospital four months later, he left his wife no debt for the hundreds of thousands of dollars the hospital charged for what would be his last stay.

America spends more on health care—both per person and in absolute dollars—than any other country, but we don't necessarily get what we pay for. We don't live as long as people in Japan, Canada, or the United Kingdom do. Despite incredibly advanced tools and treatments, not everyone gets the care he or she needs, or any care at all. Even after the politically rancorous Affordable Care Act expanded health insurance to millions of people, more than 30 million Americans remain uninsured,[1] and millions more are underinsured.[2]

"We cannot afford our health care," dozens of health care leaders across Australia told me when I traveled there in 2013 to explore high-performing health systems. "Do you know we spend 9% of our GDP on it? It's simply unsustainable." After which, some would add, "Now, why have you come *here* to learn about *our* system?" Trying to avoid creeping self-doubt that I had dragged myself across the world on a fool's errand, I would politely explain to them, and remind myself, that the United States was spending 18% of GDP on health care. I would dreamily wonder what the United States could do with an extra 9% of GDP to invest in education, infrastructure, or some other valuable part of civic life.

U.S. health care spending is not just obscene in some abstract macroeconomic sense. Each year, Americans spend nearly a trillion dollars—a number that increases every year—out of pocket on health care and health insurance. A trillion dollars is equivalent to the gross domestic product of Indonesia, a country with more than 260 million people.[3] It's a lot of money.

Even with insurance, health care costs can hurt. Approximately 158 million people get health insurance from their employer or their spouse's employer,[4] yet many are still vulnerable. The average family health plan cost more than $20,000 in 2019, 22% higher than in 2014 and 54% higher than in 2009. Employees pay more of the rising health insurance costs; 82% of employees had a deductible—compared to 63% 10 years ago—averaging approximately $1,700 per year for individuals.[5]

"We never got to a point where the insurance was paying for anything," Angela told me. A 47-year-old mother of four, she earned $22,000 a year working part-time for a nonprofit organization, while her husband got the family's health insurance through his job at a university. "We were getting it from all sides. We were paying for the premiums; we were paying the out-of-pocket; and then there was all the time involved in going to all the appointments." Angela was in physical therapy for a knee problem when they told her she needed an MRI because her condition was getting worse. Her health plan refused to pay for the MRI until she'd had an X-ray, for which she had to pay a copayment, even though she and the doctor both knew the X-ray would not be useful.

At the same time, Angela's second daughter was having recurring headaches and one night lost her balance and fell walking up the stairs. The family's pediatrician helped navigate the MRIs her daughter needed to rule out "the scary shit," which they did. And then Angela needed knee surgery, which she could not afford to pay for outright. She signed up for a payment plan with the hospital and was still a long way from paying it off when I spoke with her a year later. "I realized in the middle of all this, we had a surgery and five MRIs in our house and we didn't meet the deductible." Angela's family paid 100% of the thousands of dollars their health care cost them that season, with no help from the insurance for which they paid hundreds of dollars each month.

Angela's husband's employer had ratcheted up the family's share of health insurance costs as a mechanism for absorbing the rise in health insurance premiums, on the theory that such cost-sharing would also recruit the employees, including Angela's family, into the fight against rising costs. Surely if Angela had to pay for much of her family's care, she would judiciously avoid wasted, unnecessary care and search for lower-cost providers to stretch her own dollars. That's how the theory goes anyway.

But which of the services Angela sought were wasteful? Her daughter's symptoms could have signaled a brain tumor; should she not have pursued an immediate and thorough investigation? Wouldn't we judge her passivity if she had not, especially if something had turned out to be very wrong? When Angela's own mobility was compromised by a knee injury, should she have toughed it out? Not gotten surgery? She had gone through physical therapy, after all, trying a lower-cost, less-invasive approach first. It just didn't work for her. Angela lives in a rural state, without many choices if she's unhappy with the care or cost of her current health care providers. She felt lucky to have insurance at all, and to only pay $400 or $500 per month, when she knew too many people who were worse off.

Could Angela "shop" her way to a better result? Could Dara?

Health care is complicated. It's stressful. It's expensive. Consumers face massive disadvantages in health care encounters: we can never know more than our doctors about what we need. And that's not just a function of doctors' education; it's also a feature of the rigidly hierarchical society within which doctors operate. "Doctor knows best" is not just an old-timey phrase but the foundation of the current medical power structure. A frame of mind. A way of life. Like a con man who takes you in by making you believe, because he so obviously believes, doctors need us to trust that they know. And they need to believe they know. People's lives and health are in their hands, and lawsuits come easy, so doctors are pretty damn invested in being right. Plus, it feels good to be right.

"So-and-so is a really good doctor," I have heard so many times in my professional life and in my research. "How do you know that?" I ask. "Actually, you're right. . . . I have no idea." "They feel like a good doctor, and I want them to be, because I need them to be," might be a more honest assessment. If we are all invested in doctors being right, why would any of us upset this particular apple cart by questioning them? "Am I getting the best care from you, for the best price?" most people won't ask.

Doctors, too, feel powerless. "Insurance companies are to blame," doctors and therapists have told me over and over. My husband, a psychiatrist, used to tell me stories about phone conversations with insurance representatives, knowing they were listening for words on a checklist that could cue them to approve the hospital admission he was requesting. It wasn't hard for him to learn the key words and expertly weave them into his clinical case reports. But he objected to the charade, to wasting his time, and to being second guessed by someone without clinical training. Eventually, he stopped accepting insurance altogether, seeing some patients for free to avoid bureaucratic headaches.

For a family therapist I interviewed, taking insurance would be "like having a dictator from outside the room, orchestrating your treatments, which to me is orchestrating a relationship. And that just doesn't seem like good medicine to me." Many mental health practitioners operate outside the insurance system to avoid this dictatorship that governs treatments, timelines, and prices.

But most specialties need to operate in a larger structure—a clinic, hospital, or facility—whose lifeblood is insurance reimbursement. For most doctors, operating alone is swimming upstream; practice consolidation is common as a means of building strength, including gaining some negotiating power in their health insurance relationships. Bad medicine or not, health insurers are the third wheel in most American doctor-patient relationships.

Despite all the money flowing through the American health care system, the notion of supply and demand doesn't quite apply. Demand for health care is "irregular and unpredictable."[6] And suppliers—who clearly hold asymmetrical knowledge—are not supposed to act as salespeople, constrained by social mores to put aside their own self-interest.[7] Even as awareness grows that health care is, in fact, a business, and physician entrepreneurial urges influence health care costs,[8] American culture has not fully embraced the business of medicine.

Not surprisingly, then, the construct of a health care consumer—one who demands value from a supplier of goods or services—seems foreign. We sometimes face health care decisions at our most vulnerable moments. We often don't feel like we have any choices at all. Even if we did have choices, most of us wouldn't know how to make them. People spend more time shopping for furniture, home repairs, and even groceries. In health care, many consumers lack competence, confidence, or even the imagination to consider themselves agents in health care purchasing decisions the way we are when we spend our money on almost anything else. How, then, can we be demanding? Choosey? Entitled to value? And would it even work?

"I got a bill. A $450 bill!" the vice president of human resources brandished the envelope at me. We had been health plan executives together for many years by 2013, when this conversation occurred. "Why'd I get a bill?" My colleague's wife had gotten an MRI at a Boston teaching hospital. "You must have a deductible," I said. "Hmmm," he replied. This highly educated, seasoned professional purchased health benefits for our 500 employees, yet he did not realize that he, himself, would be out almost $500 for his wife's scan. If such a bill could take him by surprise, what chance do most people have of understanding their health benefits?

The American health care system grew up, not around individuals but around doctors, hospitals, insurance companies, public agencies, and corporations. Though until relatively recently public figures claimed the United States had "the greatest health care in the world," many Americans now recognize that the system doesn't work for everyone, at least not all the time. The biggest reform in generations—the Affordable Care Act (or Obamacare)—caused such a political stir that I had to explain it in every one of my meetings with Australian leaders. "What's the big fuss all about anyway?" asked 100% of the Australians I met, usually with a subtly—and appropriately—accusatory tone. "It doesn't even solve your whole problem."

Systemic change is not just hard because of political divisions and philosophical differences on who should provide health care to citizens. Current stakeholders have too much invested in the current setup to embrace—let alone drive—change. One man's waste is another's income. One company's opportunity is another's inefficiency, ripe for displacement. Despite entrepreneurs trying to capitalize on health care's dysfunction, for the most part, inertia—or minimal and marginal changes—reigns.

Why would making health care more shoppable be a good thing? The idea of shopping can seem frivolous—reserved for things we want, like new shoes—not things we need, like medication or surgery. Worse, shopping seems like a domain of privilege, in which people without money cannot participate. Orienting health care around shopping risks leaving those without resources behind. But evidence suggests even low-income consumers shop and have become attractive segments for some of the world's largest retailers.[9,10,11]

Shopping includes more than simply comparing prices and choosing the cheapest option, as health care experts sometimes narrowly—and dismissively—define it. Rather, shopping is shorthand for a more complex process of identifying wants and needs, determining options, evaluating those options against a wide range of criteria (as defined by the shopper), making the purchase, and evaluating how well that purchase met the original wants and needs. This process can happen unconsciously, almost instantly, such as with a simple impulse buy from the candy rack while checking out at the grocery store, or it can be explicit, methodical, even tortured, as some people engage in deep deliberation on large purchases like cars or computers.

When I need a new phone—usually because my old one has died, not because I must have the latest model—I typically start with the brand I am replacing. I look at the features and the size options. I land on a color. And I look at the price, considering if the next few megapixels in the camera are worth the extra money. I visit the store, hold it in my hand, consider paying over time or all at once—which gets harder to swallow as the prices rise, and I leave with a new phone of my choice, not necessarily the right phone or the cheapest or the newest but the one that best suits me.

Shoppers are entitled to their opinions, preferences, and priorities, whether price or convenience or brand matters most to them. They expect products that work as advertised and enjoy protections when they do not. Shopping is not reserved for wealthy people buying nonessential luxuries but is the act—by all people—of seeking what they need or want with the resources they have. Shopping, in this context, is universal. Shopping is a mind-set, a level of expectation that one deserves to have met regardless of resources or status.

Shoppers have a lot of power, more than most American health care consumers have or feel they have. Companies, and whole industries, rise and fall on consumer whims. The health care industry will not likely hand over this power voluntarily and subject itself to disruption willingly. Rather, change will need to come from consumers themselves. Consumers will need to march in the proverbial streets, raise expectations of how they should be treated, and not let up until people controlling the power structures and systems get the message.

What should consumers demand? The health policy domain is rich with possible reforms, from the dramatic to the mundane. There are obvious and ample improvement opportunities in price transparency and disclosure, access to health insurance, and standardization of benefits and consumer protections.

But Americans need only bring their indigenous consumer expertise to the table. We are native capitalists; inventors of conspicuous consumption; patrons of shopping malls, big-box stores, and all manner of online outlets. In our vast melting pot, we are connected by a common culture of consumerism. Together, we have spawned whole new industries like personal computers, smartphones, and electric cars. We have brought down crusty old systems that forced us to play by rules that worked against us; we helped democratize travel, taxis, investments, and higher education. In health care, too, we could have seismic impact. Americans should recognize rising health care costs—and our increasing share thereof—not only as burdensome financial exposure but also as potent purchasing power.

With our collective wallets, we have forced transformation in virtually every other industry. It's time for health care's turn.

1

An Ode to Shopping

How we buy everything

Our classic 1950s' Fords and Buicks—bubblegum pink and candy-shop teal, violet, and red—wind through the neighborhood. We had breezed along the Malecón, an iconic introduction to Havana's coastal locale, and disembarked temporarily at the Plaza de la Revolución. In the world's largest city square and site of many Fidel Castro political rallies, we snapped selfies under the looming steel sculpture of revolutionary hero Che Guevara affixed to the side of one government ministry building and, of course, in front of the vintage cars.

We passed imposing Soviet-era hotels, remnants of a period with even-stricter state control of the economy, in which central government agencies provided virtually the only accommodation options. Inside ugly cinderblock exteriors are relative luxuries, off limits to Cubans themselves yet insufficient to delight Americans, accustomed to bigger rooms, better plumbing, and nicer food for the price.

Today, arriving at our rented *casa particulares* (private homes or accommodations), tucked into a quiet, leafy residential neighborhood, we climb the steep steps to the patio and gratefully accept cold fruit juices from our host. We catch our breath as the airport snafu rapidly recedes. Arriving on time via a commercial flight and passing through immigration with no delays, we had entered Cuba too efficiently and caught our hosts by surprise. They hadn't even left for the airport yet, assuming it would take us hours to emerge from a bureaucratic maze. Without solid cellular service to request pickup, we had been temporarily stranded.

Now, cooling off on the terrace, it's not entirely clear whose home we are renting. How does a resident of Communist Cuba own property with rights to monetize it? Yet Airbnb took off in Havana,[1] racing to meet the demand of nearly five million tourists a year.[2] With a broader range of price points, styles, and locations—all with a local flavor—private bed and breakfasts now offer as many rooms as the state's largest conglomerate, which on its own provides one-quarter of the rooms available to international tourists.[3]

Long a forbidden destination for Americans because of U.S. law, travel restrictions had recently eased. Americans—drawn by the romance of a lingering old-world opulence in the lush tropics—are again putting Cuba on their must-see lists. Once an exotic getaway, relaxed and permissive, celebrities and high-society members had indulged in Cuba as a playground in the 1920s. Framing Cuba as the "land of romance," even the U.S. government promoted the sultry destination, emphasizing natural beauty over the casino-and-cabaret culture.[4] By the 1950s, inexpensive tour packages and proximity to Miami brought Cuba's allure down market; masses of Americans flocked to this pleasure island like they do now to Las Vegas. Despite the limitations imposed following the 1962 Cuban Missile Crisis, intrepid Americans—and plenty of Canadians and Europeans—had been undeterred from traveling to Cuba. But now, slightly less adventurous travelers could feel like explorers, investigating a bygone era while sipping *Cuba Libres* and frozen mojitos against a backdrop of palm trees, the azure Caribbean Sea, and an ever-present salsa beat.

To meet resurgent tourism demands, the private Cuban economy is thriving. In 2017, 580,000 Cubans were officially self-employed, almost three times more than a decade before. Many more work in the informal private economy. Those in tourism roles can earn more income than long-trained professionals. One tour guide described friends covering for each other's absences from government jobs while they are off trying to capture more lucrative side income. Cuba's surface-level socialism belies its innate entrepreneurial spirit, surging to meet growing demand from visitors and creating local markets at the same time. This demand has driven a boom in loving restorations of private homes, diminishing the role of aging, dark, gray, government-run hotels.

Consumerism is blossoming in the unlikeliest habitat—irrepressible and perhaps universally human.

The pedicab whizzes down Commercial Street, expertly weaving around Provincetown's summer tourists. The tourists don't always realize they are sharing the road with a range of vehicles or even with other pedestrians. The pedicab driver understands this and expertly commands the vehicle—something like a bicycle-powered rickshaw, as if the passenger seat of a horse-drawn carriage has been grafted onto a road bike. Local business advertisements are plastered to the back of the passenger seats, when they're not sporting "Just Married" signs and trailing tin cans.

The driver waves to his countless summer acquaintances on the street, like a minor celebrity or local official seeking reelection. He answers his phone, fulfilling the dispatcher's duties from the road, and tees up a fellow driver for the next pickup. At no time does he stop pedaling or navigating, until he crawls to a controlled, near-stop behind a delivery truck that is pulling to one side of the congested street to drop a package. The pedicab driver regains steam, pulling around the paused truck, and speeds on to the destination. As he pedals up the hill, his calf muscles stand out in relief, like they were carved out of stone in the image of some fictional fitness deity.

"Where are you from?" he lightly engages his passengers, turning his head so they can hear him but never losing sight of the congested landscape ahead. "First time in P-town?" he banters and asks where they've been so far, how they like it, and when they have to go home.

Slowing smoothly and angling the cart-like vehicle toward the sidewalk in front of the burger place on the opposite end of town from the departure point, the passengers begin to disembark.

"How much do we owe you?" they ask, as if to a cabdriver who'd shut off the meter.

"Whatever you feel is right," the driver replies. This thriving slice of the economy runs purely on consumers' value. The only price tag is whatever the passenger wants it to be.

A colorful bounty of vegetables arrives diagonally across the table from me, for one of my dinner companions—a vegan. We are in Indianapolis, at a steak house. Salmon and asparagus sit on a plate in front of me, steak and potatoes on one to my left.

"Even five years ago, this would not have been available," my dinner companion—a local—tells me. She wasn't vegan then but knows the evolution that has taken place in this quintessentially Midwestern, red-meat-loving capital.

Who first asked for a meal without animal products? we ponder. How strange they must have seemed, especially in an American heartland city—and the city with one of the high per capita concentrations of chain restaurants in America.[5] In the airport newsstand's souvenir magnet selection, alongside a molded tornado with a miniature house and tractor swirling in its funnel, they sell cow magnets that look like finger puppets, with "Indianapolis" quaintly stitched along the side. I interpret this to mean I am in beef country.

Where vegans used to be a fringe group on the outskirts of normal food culture, veganism has moved into the mainstream. Beyoncé, Bill Clinton, and Madonna are just some of the celebrities who have embraced veganism.[6]

"The first person seems weird," another dinner guest says. He is enjoying a steak. "But once enough people join in, it becomes widely available."

I am reminded of a video featuring a shirtless guy dancing wildly as a crowd of music-festival goers sits passively on a grassy hill around him.[7] He is unfazed, and continues dancing. The crowd around him must notice, but they sit or roam. I have no idea how long he's been dancing, but after about 20 seconds of this YouTube video, a "first follower" runs down the hill to join the dancing man[8] and dances too. They embrace, dance together, and play off each other. It takes a little more than 30 seconds before a third dancer joins them and less than 20 seconds for two more to join in. A minute and a half into the video, people are running in droves to join the group, and before the two-minute mark the dancers appear to outnumber those sitting, who are practically forced to join in or get trampled. By three minutes in, it's hard to see anyone still sitting.

Like the dancing crowd on the grassy hill, veganism is taking hold. Between 2004 and 2017, Americans identifying as vegan grew 600%, to a still relatively small 6% of the total population. As restaurants and stores recognize budding demand for vegan options, they greet that demand with additional offerings. The U.S. market for plant-based food alternatives grew 17% in one year, representing $3.7 billion in sales and far outpacing the 2% overall food sales growth.[9] By 2019, grocery sales had reached $4.5 billion for plant-based products that directly replace animal products, representing a 31% increase over two years.[10]

By now, vegan options have moved beyond coastal cafés and seem to be expanding at an accelerated pace. People for the Ethical Treatment of Animals (PETA) publishes lists of vegan-friendly chain restaurants, including Olive Garden, Cheesecake Factory, and TGI Fridays.[11] Fast-food chains like Burger King, Chipotle, Subway, and Dominos all offer legitimate vegan options.[12] In turn, more people see veganism as a viable option.

While veganism is typically grounded in concern for animals, the environment, or one's health—or some combination—consumers also make individual food choices based on taste, price, and convenience.[13] The more options available, the more plausible keeping commitments becomes. A once-lonely stance becomes accepted. The sole guy dancing shifts from loner to leader. Similarly, social norms that might suppress one's willingness to persist in a vegan lifestyle give way to tolerance, embrace, and influence. I find myself easily convinced by my dinner companion's arguments in favor of veganism, my own guilt already bubbling up about cruelty to animals and care for the planet and my own body. Whether I have the will of my new friend is quite another matter, but I feel no urge to deny or fight her position. I feel only respect.

And like that, the movement migrates from the margins to the mainstream.

Consumer preferences, tastes, and tolerances emerge and evolve, and nudge cultural norms—and consumer markets—forward. The not-so-underground Cuban capitalism responding to new demand, the Province-town pedicabs, and the mainstreaming of plant-based diets are just a few examples of how consumer purchasing power takes hold of markets and shapes how people access and consume goods and services.

There are many more.

Blockbuster fell to Netflix, and then Netflix disrupted its own disc mail-in service as streaming technology improved.

Expedia, Kayak, and dozens more online travel sites made travel agents, paper tickets, and printed itineraries a set of relics from another time, more recent than the golden age of travel but every bit as defunct.

Amazon gobbled up all the bookstores and more, and gave rise to a countermovement to "shop local" in support of small proprietors.

Uber sent taxi companies into protectionism mode, only delaying the inevitable spread of efficient, flexible, fairly reliable, ride-hailing apps. Early in my career, I worked for someone who called two taxis as a rule, figuring one would inevitably not show up. "You're the reason they don't show up," I pointed out the circularity and potential impact of his own no-show rate. If people aren't reliably waiting for the taxi they've called, taxi drivers won't be as reliable in picking up passengers. In turn, because taxis are some-times unreliable, some passengers like my colleague call two, guaranteeing someone is left waiting for a no-show. The lack of visibility and account-ability on both sides illustrates why Uber holds so much obvious appeal for both drivers and riders.

Consumer purchasing power can create new categories, anointing win-ners as new options appear.

So, too, can consumers undo inferior products, companies, and whole categories. We can no longer visit a big-box store to rent a movie. If you want help from a person when planning your travel, it will be hard to secure. Beef isn't dead, but U.S. consumption is definitely on the decline.[14]

In the early 1990s, a small group of angry consumers used their collec-tive voice to hold a major consumer products company to account. As reported by Zachary Crockett in *The Hustle* in August 2019,[15] Hoover vac-uums had been a household name in the United Kingdom, the brand syn-onymous with the category, like Kleenex and Band-Aid. However, by the late 1980s, this most trusted brand—which had been acquired by Maytag—was bumping up against both competition from innovators like Dyson and a recession in Britain. Profits fell by half between 1987 and 1992, and its dominant market share began to erode.

Desperate to regain ground, Hoover launched a Hail Mary marketing promotion late in 1992. Buy a Hoover product of at least £100 and get two free tickets from the United Kingdom to the United States. Surely, consumers would buy more than £100 worth of goods, and few would actually collect the airplane tickets. The whole theory of rebates, where you get a great price *if* you mail something to the corporation within a certain amount of time, works on the premise that most people do not follow through. The theory usually holds true.

This time, it did not. On £30 million of vacuum sales—the average value of which was not significantly more than the £100 threshold—Hoover accrued at least £100 million of liability for the promised free tickets.

Facing huge potential financial losses, the company started jilting consumer attempts to redeem the flights. They allegedly pretended to lose entries, timed mailings to decrease redemptions, and offered itineraries so unattractive that consumers would hopefully abandon their claims. When consumers caught wind of these deliberate sabotage attempts, they went for the company's jugular. An angry consumer coalition of just 4,000 people—though hundreds of thousands were affected—demanded the company honor its promotion.

Eventually, Maytag paid more than $70 million for 220,000 customers' flights, leaving many more customers without ever getting their due. By the end of 1993, Hoover had accumulated a 6% net loss. In 1995, Maytag sold the Hoover division at a loss, and the company's market share fell from 50% to 10%. Hoover products were rated "least reliable," and the company's reputation hit bottom.

Consumers give, and consumers take away.

Purchasing power gives rise to categories, companies, and products that meet consumer needs and preferences. Consumers reward companies that offer meaningfully better service, lower prices, or novel solutions.

Consumers can also use economic power to send strong signals to the market about what they will tolerate. In this way, consumers can force powerful corporations to deliver value, and punish products and approaches that don't work, simply by moving their money elsewhere or—in extreme cases like Hoover—by pulling out all the stops and shaming the entities that fail to deliver.

The Hoover case is a cautionary tale for marketers and corporations, in general. You can't pretend to offer consumers false value and get away with it. Like dogs who sense fear and children who intuit adult emotions, consumers will sniff that out and vote with their wallets.

Hoover is also a reminder to consumers: when companies fail to deliver value, or falter on their promises, it is possible to hold them accountable. Being unwilling to tolerate fraud, injustice, or simply inefficiency is the first step, and speaking up about it or joining others' campaigns for value can make the difference.

In the positive, when consumers band together, aggregate spending can make a huge impact. Just as American diners are spawning more plant-based options, Americans can inspire a better, more responsive, higher-value health system.

Sam Walton reportedly said, "There is only one boss. The customer. And he can fire everybody in the company from the chairman on down, simply by spending his money elsewhere."[16] Sam Walton's ethos shows a healthy respect for the power of American wallets.

Let that be a battle cry for health care consumers everywhere.

2

This Is Not Nordstrom

How American health care fails consumers

Jessica stood behind the counter in the second-floor dress department of a high-end retailer. She had a phone to one ear and an eye on the situation in front of her. An anxious woman holding a long purple dress stood alongside her teen daughter. The mom was intently focused on Jessica and the answer they were both awaiting from the other end of the phone. The girl was at least as tall as her mother, with long, straight, light-brown hair. The purple prom gown would strikingly complement her fair skin. It seemed like a simple, perhaps slinky dress with spaghetti straps and a touch of bedazzle on the bodice. But for the color—a bright, confident purple in the grape soda family—it might have been almost understated. Something seemed to have gone wrong in alterations. The mother-daughter pair had gone back to the dressing room to try it one more time, but they had returned to confirm it was just not right.

Jessica exuded the energy of a seasoned sea captain steering a ship about to go off course or an athletic person balancing his or her weight on a paddle board in stronger-than-typical waves. She projected a steady yet high-intensity determination to master a difficult situation. I could almost see her tick through a mental library of potential contingency plans as she waited for what she hoped would be the simplest one—a replacement dress that could be rush-shipped in time for this girl's prom.

When the call did not end well—the right dress in the right size seemed out of stock across the chain—Jessica took action. She had called in a manager—a thin man in an elegant black suit—who was now taking down the mother's information and confirming the store stood firmly behind Jessica's approach. The mother had located the dress elsewhere online, and I imagine the resolution had something to do with reimbursement for the new dress and certainly a refund for the faultily tailored one. I didn't track the specifics but noticed the mother's energy had shifted from edgy to resigned, and I was surprised that no one appeared furious, and no one was crying. The mother graciously thanked Jessica as she and her daughter left.

From my place in line, I watched this scene with a small pit in my stomach. The saleswoman who was trying to help me find the dress I had bought the week before seemed nervous. I had left it for alterations so it could be ready for an event coming up in two weeks. The saleswoman had looked for my dress and returned empty handed. She had waited her turn to get Jessica's input—which Jessica gave efficiently in the midst of her prom-gown-gone-awry salvage attempts.

They finally found my dress in a different department, but my own dress's alterations were also not quite right. Too long in some places and too short in others, the flouncy hem of the layered long dress was irreparable, deemed the on-duty seamstress. They should get me a new one and try again, except this store did not have one in stock.

When it was my turn with Jessica, I had no doubt, based on what I had just witnessed, that she and the store she represented would make it work.

DEFINING HEALTH CARE PURCHASING

"What's a health care purchase?"

When I first started interviewing consumers for my study on health care consumer behavior, I opened each interview asking participants to generate a list of some recent health care purchases they had made. My goal was to understand what prevents—and what could enable—individuals from behaving in health care as they typically do in other categories: as shoppers who use their purchasing power, however large or small, to signal their preferences, needs, and priorities to the market. If I could understand how people make and feel about specific financial decisions in health care, I could test industry assumptions that consumers do not—and maybe cannot—shop in a health care context and shed light on the key ingredients of a more effective consumer health care market.

"What's a health care purchase?" one participant asked in response to the seemingly simple prompt. Though I had tried to avoid health care jargon by using plain English, it became clear that the question was confusing people. Assuming I had not formed a very good question, I initially jumped in with an explanation. "You know, any time you spend your own money on anything to do with your health care or coverage," I would explain.

After a few interviews, I realized that even if I was asking a poorly formed question, the confusion about it was, itself, telling.

What part of "purchase" didn't people understand? Purchasing is defined as "acquisition of (something) by paying for it." Simply, it's buying something. What more straightforward a concept could I use to find out how people decide how to spend their health care dollars?

I felt a little mean when I stopped explaining the question, just to see what people came up with, because many people flailed.

"Can you tell us about some health care purchases you've made?" I asked Clara, a 98-year-old great grandmother.

"Health? I didn't quite get that." This is where I felt mean. "Health care purchases?" she asked again after I repeated the question. "I don't know that area. What purchases?"

I asked the same question of Sam, another retiree. "I'm sorry, say that again?" He stumbled even after he clearly heard the question, "Health care purchases. I'm not sure what qualifies."

One of my research assistants asked a young woman, Alexa, to talk about her health care purchases. "What does that mean?" she asked for clarification. "I literally have no idea what you're talking about."

The first finding from these interviews may seem obvious: people do not consciously connect notions of shopping to their health care decisions. In health care, it is foreign to think about the money we spend as anything resembling a purchase. What might the impact be if consumers recognized themselves as health care purchasers?

Beyond terminology, there was a deeper disconnect. Leah, a mom in her 40s fighting an ovarian cancer recurrence, summed up why spending money on health care did not feel like purchasing. "I have to do it. It's not optional," she described her monthly or every-other-month hospital visits for cancer checks. "To me, a purchase is more like, I want these higher-heeled shoes for my bursitis. That is a purchase. Something that's a little more discretionary. Whereas if I don't get the CT scan, I might miss a tumor that is growing and it's going to kill me and I'll die. . . . It doesn't feel like a purchase to me, it just feels like something I have to do."

The dire stakes cause economists to question the viability of consumer shopping for health care: if you have to get it—as in emergency or medically necessary care—it's not something you can shop for. It's just not a purchase.

For Amanda, a young professional, services relating to an emergency room encounter "don't jump to mind when I think about purchasing, even though I paid for them, because it was an emergent situation. It wasn't elective." Reflecting on her emergency experience, though, she realized several points where she was presented with options or made choices, many with financial implications. "I do think there's this huge divide between the emergent situations and the chronic conditions, even though there were all these purchasing decisions that I didn't realize until now with the emergency."

More commonly, people thought about health care purchases in literal terms. For example, Nicole, a graduate student, ventured an idea. "Purchases? Like over-the-counter medication kind of stuff?" Eric, another young adult, also defined purchases in an over-the-counter context. "Sudafed," he said but wanted to be sure. "Does that count?"

Lillian, a semiretired nurse on Medicare, also thought of supplements or other over-the-counter items; to her, a health care purchase was something for which "you don't need to access a health care provider."

Some consumers naturally connected the idea of spending money to health insurance, particularly insurance that they bought themselves. Gregg, who bought individual insurance on the ACA marketplace, thought about his health plan selection and the health care spending that occurs out of pocket. "When you say health care purchases, are you talking about insurance or outside of insurance?"

Hazel, a graphic designer and small-business owner, also saw the link to insurance. "Something outside of just picking a health insurance plan, like it's a surgery or something like that?"

Consumers with high-deductible plans recognized their out-of-pocket responsibilities as purchasing. "Almost by definition everything we do is purchased, because we have a high-deductible plan," said George, a finance professional in the New York City area. He was well aware of his family's health care spending.

Rosemary, a stay-at-home mom of two, similarly felt the impact of her deductible. "We have to meet our deductible before anything is really covered. I think it's a thousand-dollar deductible, so we hit that pretty fast." She took me through a litany of health care services her family has had to pay for: mental health counseling, EpiPens for her daughter who is allergic to "a million things," and gap insurance coverage via COBRA* when her husband was in between jobs. "There's a lot of things our insurance doesn't cover that we have to pay for," she said.

"Certainly some of these tests I got felt like big purchases," Sean said of a recent health care encounter. His primary care doctor had referred him

* The Consolidated Omnibus Budget Reconciliation Act allows employees to buy their employer's health insurance even after terminating employment.

for an MRI in the same hospital system where the physician practiced. "I have to say I was not particularly an active consumer in doing that. . . . I just went with that and I guess I definitely should have looked into if there was a lower-cost option. But I figured that it was so hard for me to have any idea to judge quality versus costs, and that it's where my doctor was recommending, they were going to have all my information, it was within the same hospital system, and so I went with that."

Undergoing treatment for pancreatic cancer, Andrea had extensive health care experience. "I've had hospital visits. I've had a lot of CT scans. I've been on lots of different medications, chemotherapy. I've had surgeries recently," she described an array of services she needed, some of which she paid for out of pocket. She was one of few consumers I interviewed who had no problem understanding the idea of purchasing in health care. For her, though, the concept of purchasing did not match the gravity of her situation. "You don't want to just be a consumer; you need to be more of an advocate for yourself and really think about how these drugs are going to impact your health. You need to be more aware than you normally are when you're purchasing things."

Unlike Andrea, who thought health care purchasing deserves more attention, many people invested less in health care decisions than in other purchases.

"Is there some kind of product that you would really do your homework before you bought it?" Anna Ford, my research collaborator, asked Bella, a young woman who had recently bought her own health insurance for the first time. Bella paused. "I feel like I pay attention to which grocery stores have better prices on granola bars." She mocked herself a bit. "I go to [a] different grocery store to save 30 cents on granola bars."

A QUESTION-LESS HEALTH CARE CONSUMER

My stomach starts to feel warm, from the inside. The slow burn develops and starts to feel like someone has taken a hot quarter and seared my stomach lining with it like a rancher might brand his or her cattle. That pain diffuses, making its way around my whole stomach.

The first time this happened, I had just eaten a piece of Italian-style strata, an egg dish with loads of vegetables, including onions, and red and green peppers. My stomach had started to burn, and eventually I had to lie down with sharp pains.

After multiple doctor visits and tests to rule out an ulcer or worse, my doctor basically put her hands up in defeat. "We could call it an allergy," she suggested but offered no cure.

I visited an acupuncturist who felt confident he could fix what he assumed was stress-induced "CEO stomach," as he called it. Acupuncture improved musculoskeletal aches but not my stomach, so the acupuncturist prescribed herbs. "Mix a tablespoon of this into hot water four times a day until the bottle is done," he advised. I paid $20 for the bottle and left, armed with my marching orders.

The "tea" was truly disgusting, its bitterness searing as I reluctantly let it travel down my throat. But if it would fix my stomach, it was worth it.

"What's that stuff supposed to do?" my husband asked when he watched me cringe through the first dose.

"Actually," I told him, "I have no idea."

If I could so blindly follow the recommendation of a caregiver I trusted, though not even a medical professional, I should not be surprised at how rarely consumers I interviewed described feeling like empowered health care shoppers. I exhibited no such empowerment—I hadn't asked about the risks, alternatives, or cost before paying—in a relatively low-stakes situation. In fact, I had not asked a single question.

BARRIERS TO HEALTH CARE SHOPPING

Americans spend approximately $1 trillion each year out of pocket on health care and coverage, about one-third of all health care spending in the United States.[1,2] That's just a bit more than what consumers spend during a typical Christmas shopping season each year.[3] Retailers organize themselves around massive holiday-season spending, wooing those dollars through advertising and promotions, extended hours, and extra staff. Many holiday shoppers lose their heads, slaves to long wish lists or caught up in the spirit of the season. Many carry credit card balances and pay steeply in January and beyond. But all drive their own purchases.

Despite comparable spending out of consumers' pockets each year, health care works differently for many reasons. Here are seven commonly cited obstacles to health care shopping:

1. **Information asymmetry:** Consumers can never know as much about health and health care as their health care providers. Doctors go to four years of medical school and continue their training in residency for three to seven years. Many who specialize complete additional training in fellowships. To get on this track in the first place, premedical college students must master organic chemistry and a battery of other rigorous science courses. They pass a grueling standardized test—the Medical College Admission Test®—and invest in an involved application and interview process. By the time they become doctors, this group has proven their intellect, their determination, and their commitment. They deserve a lot of the deference they get.

And many consumers don't *want* to know that much, an attitude Ruby—a high school teacher—epitomized. "It's an area where I feel a bit at a loss," she said. Looking for a new doctor tripped her up. "Where do I start? I don't know the questions to ask. I'm not a doctor. If I have to know what questions to ask, that's a problem to me." She sought doctors who would guide her. "Is it someone who will be able to walk me through and help me see the questions I didn't know to ask?"

2. **Complexity:** Medicine itself has become too complex for any human to know fully. Doctors themselves—high-performing professionals prepared by a lifetime of training—often struggle to keep pace with scientific discoveries and clinical best practices. At Harvard Medical School, the New Pathway curriculum was developed in 1987[4] as a problem-based approach, recognizing the need to train physicians to find answers—rather than to memorize answers—because although the right answer would change over time a problem-solving mind-set could persist across generations of discovery and new means of accessing information.

Still, the average time for a discovery to become standard in clinical practice is generally accepted to be 17 years,[5] about equivalent to the half-life of an average physician's career. The implication is that doctors practice as they are trained, and only after a new generation of physicians replaces them do newer approaches enter mainstream medicine.

Dr. Michael Ostacher, professor of psychiatry and behavioral sciences at Stanford Medical School and digital content editor for the journal *Evidence-Based Mental Health,* explained why it is so hard for doctors to keep up with the volume of new scientific evidence. "It's a time thing," he told me. People "tend to only read the abstracts of papers or they tend to only listen to key opinion leaders about what they should do, rather than being critical themselves about the evidence." Financial incentives don't help, he explained. "You're not paid to keep up with the information. You're paid to treat your patients. So, you have to do this in time that you're not getting paid for, and for some people that's really a concern. It's usually reading at night in extra hours. And you know, I'd rather watch a soccer match and make dinner for my family, frankly."

Much-hyped artificial intelligence promises to help bring order to vast quantities of health care data. Just as such advances may help physicians manage complexity, consumers may also benefit from decision aids based on these methods. Right answers may become more knowable through sophisticated algorithms and analyses.

In the meantime, many health care decisions involve complex information, which many consumers are simply not equipped to understand or access. Health care and health insurance each have their own languages, rules, and processes. If you're not an insider, it can be as difficult to navigate as the subway map when a non-Japanese-speaking visitor first arrives in Tokyo. Actually, the Tokyo subway system follows some order, and novices can study and learn it. Yet even health care insiders admit they are often confused by bureaucratic intricacies. Chapters 11 and 12 delve into the impact of complexity in health insurance.

How could consumers, even engaged and educated ones, possibly keep up?

3. **Price opacity:** Despite price transparency laws and tools, it remains extremely difficult to find health care prices. Difficulty predicting what services will be needed further complicates price transparency. The nuances of different insurance rules applied to different services in different settings make exposing prices truly challenging.

Many consumers report wanting to engage in cost conversations with their doctors but not getting to do so.[6] Still others are uncomfortable, afraid, or simply don't think to ask the price. Doctors and other health professionals may not even know what the price is if a consumer does ask. Where price transparency tools are available to doctors, adoption can be slow. Humana's drug pricing tool, for example, had less than 10% adoption in 2019 despite being available since 2015.[7] Chapter 5 explores the root causes of price opacity and the potential of price transparency.

4. **Vulnerability and sensitivity:** Consumers face many health care decisions under emotional duress or strain, when the stakes are high, sometimes even a matter of life and death. It is difficult to shop around under those conditions. Research shows that people under stress do not make optimal decisions. In some studies, participants made decisions too quickly, without fully assessing alternatives; in others, participants made riskier decisions which more often led to worse outcomes.[8] Risk-averse health insurance decisions can lead consumers to opt—and have to pay—for more coverage than they need.[9] And consumers under stress may not fully process their treatment options, resulting in suboptimal care decisions. Vulnerable consumers may be least able to advocate for themselves.

In Chapter 8, I share Amanda's story about an emergency in which clinicians insisted on conducting tests she argued were unnecessary; she had just had many of them done at a regular checkup not long before. "I was writhing in pain on the table," she told me. "I wasn't going to fight tooth and nail to skip these tests, but I made it very clear that it was not necessary and that I did not want to do them." Who knows if the treating clinicians would have listened to her had she been well, but she certainly was not in the best position to insist on being heard.

5. **Power asymmetry:** Information asymmetry, complexity, and vulnerability all contribute to an imbalance of power. Doctors tend to tell patients what to do, and patients tend to almost blindly follow, according to Heather Ross, PhD, DNP, ANP-BC, clinical assistant professor at the Arizona State University Edson College of Nursing and Health Innovation and School for the Future of Innovation in Society.

    "It's not just an information asymmetry. It *is* an information asymmetry, but it translates to a power asymmetry, wherein people don't feel empowered to make choices like that between different conditions or different settings. They just make the choice to, 'Yes, fill the prescription,' or 'No, don't fill the prescription.'" Instead of asking for alternatives, many patients simply avoid taking the prescription she has written if they cannot afford it. They would rather quietly go without recommended care than openly expose their financial strain or question their provider. Scared, uncomfortable, suffering, or simply not in charge of the situation—consumers in many health care encounters are not on equal footing with the professionals caring for them.

6. **Consumer incentives:** "People who shop don't matter economically, and people who matter economically don't shop," Bob Kocher, MD,[10] told me in an interview. A notable health care venture capitalist and one of the shapers of the Affordable Health Care Act as a member of the Obama administration, he questioned the fundamental premise and potential impact of health care shopping.

    In effect, he made a case against the reality and potential of health care shopping. His point is that the people who use the most health care services and cost the system the most tend to rapidly satisfy their deductible and exceed their out-of-pocket spending limits. At that point, most of their care is presumably fully covered by insurance, so these consumers become shielded from any financial incentive to shop around or use services more judiciously. These costly people matter because together they represent a huge proportion of overall health care costs, but they are not paying for most of it themselves. Once they have paid their share, they have little reason to shop beyond, perhaps, researching quality of care.

    Conversely, if someone does not meet their deductible, by definition, that person is likely not using a lot of services. He or she may be more sensitive to the costs of care, but to the overall system, those costs are relatively insignificant. The cost of high utilizers dwarfs any savings lower utilizers might achieve by shopping. Thus, the people with the incentive to shop—those who are on the hook for their own health care spending—just do not matter when it comes to bending the cost curve.

7. **Industry incentives:** The concept of consumerism is that if individuals take charge of their health care, shop around, and vote with their feet and their wallets, then the industry will need to respond with lower costs and better, more consumer-oriented service and product options. But health care is a $3.5 trillion industry. That isn't just a lot of spending; it's a lot of revenue for health care organizations. Rarely do companies or other institutions willingly give up revenue or do anything to put their financial results in jeopardy. They cling to power and fight disruption. If increasing transparency or "shoppability" redistributes value to favor consumers, then health care institutions stand to lose. Thus, industry financial incentives favor the status quo, and incumbent players will resist the transformation to a consumer-grade health care system.

Despite these barriers to consumer health care shopping, consumer incentives are shifting, as are behaviors. People are trying to become more educated health care consumers. Half of Americans report trying to find out how much they will have to pay out of pocket before getting care; people with deductibles greater than $3,000 and people without insurance are more likely to seek price information. Nearly three-quarters of people in one survey felt their doctors or their staff should discuss price with them before they order tests or procedures, yet less than one-third reported having had these conversations. This information can affect behavior and positively impact costs overall; more than half of those who have tried to compare prices chose less expensive care.[11] That those cost savings reduce revenue for someone may help explain why those conversations are so rare.

The American health care system is simply not built around consumers the way other consumer markets are. "I just wanted it to be easy," Margaret told me. A marketing professional working in the field, she is not a typical health care consumer. Still, she experienced a frustrating billing situation in which a provider was billing inconsistent amounts, and she had wound up over- or underpaying. "I wanted to be able to make one phone call and have it all sorted." That wasn't her experience, as she had to toggle between the health plan and the provider, caught in between. "You run into people who are not that competent, who don't really understand, and they can't solve your problem, nor do they seem to really care about solving your problems. If I ordered [something] from Amazon or Nordstrom, they're going to immediately make sure I get my money and see what I was supposed to be charged and make adjustments. And you don't get that level of customer service in the health care space."

CUSTOMER OBSESSION

According to lore,[12] a customer once walked into a Nordstrom store seeking to return a pair of tires. Founded as a shoe store in 1901, Nordstrom never sold tires. Nevertheless, the staff person reportedly processed the return, and the legend of Nordstrom's flexible return policy was etched into the company's brand.

After my own department store experience—that had veered toward the edge of terrible only to be salvaged by a great salesperson—I was curious how great retailers deliver consistently good customer service across complex operations staffed by large and distributed workforces. Could their techniques apply to health care organizations?

I approached Jessica, the dress saleswoman, for her perspective and learned that her own brand of customer service did not originate with her employer. She came to her job already "prepackaged" as a service professional extraordinaire. A fourth-generation salesperson, her grandmother owned a dress shop, where her mother also worked. "I learned how to make all of these people happy, I'm not exaggerating when I say from birth." When she left the hospital as a newborn, she was "put into a laundry basket and taken to the shop."

Jessica learned an old-school model of customer service based on relationships built over many years of patronage. "You don't really find it anymore," she said. When buying merchandise from designers, Jessica's mother and grandmother would pick specific dresses in specific colors and sizes with specific customers in mind. "That's how well they knew [their customers]."

The number-one skill Jessica brought to her retail job? "I know how to listen." When she first meets a customer, she asks them a lot of questions. What is the event you're shopping for? Where is it? How dressy is it? Before they even start talking about clothes at all, Jessica first seeks to understand the customer's need, to get a picture of the event in her mind and filter out garments she knows will not work.

"People don't like to shop for dresses," Jessica said, which surprised me, because I love shopping for dresses. "It's a crowded marketplace," she further explained. "[Customers] have no idea. They're unfamiliar with the product. They show up, their blood pressure's through the roof. They don't know what's going on."

That sounded familiar, like how patients can feel when trying to get an appointment with a new doctor or navigating complex health care decisions. Health care consumers are often stressed out. We don't necessarily understand the system, the lingo, the "product." Consumers have a disadvantage given our relative knowledge. But a professional like Jessica can fast-forward to a great option—and often puts customers directly into the dress they leave with. In contrast, customers have to sort through dozens or more possibilities to find the right one. I wondered who could play that role for us in health care settings.

Jessica imbued the shopping process with more weight and meaning than I think most dress shoppers may recognize. To her, shopping is not a frivolous, optional pastime but a high-stakes endeavor to fulfill a personal need. Preparing for an important life event, feeling good about one's self, presenting one's self to the world appropriately and confidently—not frivolous at all.

The essence of Jessica's approach boils down to empowerment—of customers and staff.

"We trust our customers," Jessica explained. "We're going to assume that we can do right by them. We assume that they're trying to do right by us. And that's the basic tenet where we start." This mentality explains why it's so easy to return things to most large retailers; ease of returns in turn makes it easier to buy things. Jessica follows her company's rules and policies, but she boiled down her approach to returns this way: "Just be a good human."

I once mistakenly ordered two copies of the same book from Amazon. When I tried to return one, they told me just to keep it and refunded my purchase anyway. Amazon's administrative efficiency outweighed the cost of my refund. Their calculus also left an unquantifiable positive impression on me. Amazon cared more about the experience—mine and theirs—than about the last dollar to which they were entitled.

Jessica also explained that her employer encourages her to use good judgment to solve customer problems, whatever they might be. Like the solution to the purple prom gown or my own alterations gone awry, Jessica has autonomy to figure out solutions. "We were empowered. We could solve it on the fly," which makes customers really happy. I asked if she had ever gotten in trouble for any of her independent judgments to resolve customer issues. On the contrary, she has won an award recognizing her outstanding service.

Jessica's central philosophy coalesces as customer obsession, which manifests with a consistent effort at a starting gate: "Build the connection, figure out what the need is. Why are they here? How can I help?" She focuses not on the biggest sale or the most sales but on meeting customer needs. "I'd rather make a clean sale where I know you're going to look good. You're going to feel good. Did I sell you the most expensive thing? Maybe, maybe not. But are you going to tell all your friends to come see me? Yeah."

And it works. Jessica consistently performs in the top tier of salespeople. She is very effective at her job.

Still, Jessica questioned, "What is the business case for kindness?" She delights in performing well but is intrinsically motivated by deeper societal forces. "Some of the questions I ask myself [are] where has the connection gone? Where's the grace? Where's the common sense, and where along the way did we lose the idea that we, the company, the entity, the corporation trumps everybody else in the exchange, in the transaction, in the enterprise, when, at the end of the day, it's people who are making up the transactions."

HOSPITALITY INTELLIGENCE

I heard part of the case for kindness during the summer of 2019 at the Healthcare Thinkathon organized by the Center for Healthcare Innovation and Implementation Sciences at Indiana University's School of Medicine. There, I met Professor Godwin-Charles Ogbeide. A scholar who studies hospitality competencies and strategies, Ogbeide captivated a room full of health care leaders with his booming voice, giant personality, and sense of humor. His framework—coined "hospitality intelligence"[13]—deconstructs critical components of highly effective customer service experiences and serves as a guide for individuals and organizations seeking to bring to life the values and principles into which Jessica was born.

"Hospitality intelligence is the ability to deliberately attend to people with friendliness, empathy, and kindness," Ogbeide emphasized.

Ogbeide's framework includes seven dimensions: (1) enthusiasm, (2) acknowledgment, (3) friendliness, (4) respect, (5) empathy, (6) kindness, and (7) gratitude. This type of intelligence is learnable, Ogbeide told me, "but you have to want to learn it."

You also have to mean it. "When I say deliberately, I'm not saying fake it," he told the engaged Thinkathon crowd. "No!" he bellowed. "It has to come from within you." I asked him if you can teach that kind of authenticity. "It is hard to teach people to mean it," he said. "Meaning it comes from you. But you can inspire people to mean it, by giving them a reason to believe in it."

Jessica means it. She defines her retail role in terms that go far beyond how people often think about shopping for clothes. "Most people walk through their life and . . . no one feels appreciated. No one feels seen. No one feels heard. If you see someone, you hear someone, you connect with them . . . you [can] have a conversation that changes everything." Despite her concrete sales accomplishments, it's in these terms that Jessica measures the "business case for the kindness, for the connection, for having the empathy, for caring."

SHOPPING FOR HEALTH CARE

What would health care look like if it were a true consumer market? If health care organizations behaved more like Amazon and Nordstrom, and less like the Department of Motor Vehicles or the IRS? If all health care workers and leaders studied and implemented Ogbeide's hospitality model? If Jessica's approach and mentality were the norm? And if consumers felt heard, seen, connected, and accompanied in their journeys by someone who cares?

The rest of this book illustrates what such a system could look like. In contrast to what people experience today, the chapters that follow outline what consumers should expect and demand in exchange for their health care dollars. This book suggests a path that could help catalyze the systemic change needed to make American health care work better for the people paying for it: increasingly, consumers themselves.

3

How Does That Make You Feel?

How psychotherapy functions as a free
market and what we can learn from it

"I basically chose my psychiatrist off of the Internet," Theo told me.
A 40-year-old freelance writer and film producer based in Los Angeles, he
cited two reasons for his pick. "One, he was covered in my network, and
two, he was in walking distance to my apartment."

Theo chose his psychiatrist like he might find a restaurant or dry cleaner,
and the process worked for him. "I liked him immediately," Theo said. During that first year, he saw the psychiatrist once or twice a week while they
tried different combinations of medication for major depression and attention deficit-hyperactivity disorder (ADHD). The depression medication
was relatively easy, but everything for ADHD made Theo feel terrible.
Eventually, they landed on a medication that "didn't make me feel as weird
and bad as the others." Theo's insurance plan covered the medications with
$15 copayments. For another $40 copayment per visit, Theo had basically
unlimited coverage. The costs added up, but Theo found it affordable.

Skeptics have long believed consumers cannot, and perhaps should not,
be expected to shop for health care. Health care is too different a category
from others on which consumers spend money. The knowledge required is
too specialized, and the myriad obstacles outlined in Chapter 2 make it
near impossible.

But in mental health care—psychotherapy specifically—consumers already act like customers. Market forces drive both supply and demand. Therapy patients evaluate their options, search for best-fit solutions, and vote with their wallets. They recognize their role as purchasers and trade off costs and benefits like they might when buying other consumer goods or services. Though it can be hard to "break up" with a therapist, as I described in the Introduction, people do leave therapists who don't fit their needs, sensing that they are entitled to a therapist who does. After all, in many cases, they're paying for that service. It should work for them.

Consumers often drive mental health purchasing out of necessity: only 55% of psychiatrists accept insurance (compared with 89% of physicians in other specialties),[1] so many consumers who need care must pay out of pocket. They often have to call multiple clinicians before finding one who can see them. The financial and logistical burdens can make mental health care inaccessible for many who need it, while also illustrating the presence of market forces in mental health care.

Providers are often direct suppliers of mental health care. They set rates and rules of engagement, discuss costs, and even negotiate. Unlike clinicians who practice deep in the bowels of complex health care bureaucracies—largely shielded from direct exposure to economic elements of practice—therapists are often frontline players. Commonly solo practitioners or working in small groups, they receive direct consumer signals about price, quality, and satisfaction.

These market forces behind psychotherapy unfolded before Theo's eyes. "I think I might have been one of four clients at the beginning," he reflected. The setting was modest, a shared rented office with the entrance through the back and no receptionist. The practice was a small business just getting started. "I really liked him and that he was really helping me, and he was really, really, really smart, and he was just young."

Over time, Theo noticed changes. "I slowly got the sense that he was building his business." The adjacent offices were now occupied by 10 full-time psychiatrists who had joined the practice, working in a huge suite on two renovated floors. Theo observed four staff members and a new Internet portal. "Now he's doing his second location. He stopped seeing me personally two years ago."

The doctor's gains were Theo's loss. "He runs his business," Theo explained. "Why would he see me anymore? He's basically a business owner, and very, very, very successful."

Theo moved on to another psychiatrist in the practice and then to another after that one left. Theo viewed his current psychiatrist—a pharmacologist—as a technician. "He's basically a drug dealer. I go to him, he asks me how I'm doing. I'm like, 'The same.' He says, 'Do you need a higher dosage?' I say 'No,' and he sends me out to buy my drugs."

Where Theo used to have what felt like a relationship, his mental health care became transactional. "It is just like an oil change. I go into this place, now every three months because that's about as long as he can prescribe these things for. As soon as I'm going to run out of the last refill, I go and see him again. It's not really helpful in any way except continuing."

Theo could have gone elsewhere, but he chose to stay with the practice because he gets what he needs. "The only way I can function is on these medications. I make light of it but I'm not going to stop taking these medications because I feel like it's bullshit. They help me, but it's hysterical, I see my doctor for five minutes." This market, strange as it is, works for Theo.

In contrast, Colette's therapy encounters are far from transactional. "[My therapist] knows me better than anyone else," Colette said. One of many consumers who pay for psychotherapy out of pocket, she plans to "continue always as long as this woman is alive."

Colette had begun therapy in her 20s but had had "unhelpful experiences." Still, she remained interested in psychology and felt she would benefit from a good therapist.

When her marriage began crumbling, she found herself in crisis. Her colleague recommended a therapist who was covered by their employee health plan. Colette pursued the support she felt she desperately needed.

"It wasn't great at first," Colette reflected. "It was hard work, but I trusted her. Because she's trained as a social worker, she actually was giving me very useful immediate crisis-control resolution." Over time, their relationship strengthened and became invaluable. "I'm going to pay anything to stay in that relationship."

Colette's willingness to pay was tested first when her therapist stopped taking her insurance. Still employed and married at that time, Colette could afford the session costs. But when Colette lost her job and finalized her divorce, the fees became a hardship. "I wasn't sure how I was going to do it." She spoke openly about finances with her therapist. "She knows I can't afford much. If there's a bad month, I don't pay her until after that month. She makes it possible for me." Colette manages her visits to make sure she gets what she needs but in an affordable way for her situation. "If I'm having to be cautious with money, I'll see her once every three weeks. And [it's] still very useful. I would not stop it."

CONSUMERS IN THE DRIVER'S SEAT

On the demand side of this market, consumers who pay for their own mental health care feel like the purchaser, in charge of the decisions about their mental health care needs.

"It's more like I'm buying a consumer service," said Margaret, who was paying $75 per session out of pocket. Her therapist's full rate was $150, and it felt unreasonable to expect a discount steeper than 50%. Still, she had to weigh the costs against the benefits. "It's about expectations of value. Do I get what I need? Yes, but if I didn't, I'd be pissed. That's a very consumer-style behavior to have expectations like that."

For many consumers, mental health treatment is vital; others make trade-offs based on their budgets. Sophie described rationing the 30 visits her insurance covered and discontinuing sessions when she used those up.

For Ruby, psychotherapy was a service to be weighed against others. "It was therapy or the gym," she couldn't afford both. "I picked the gym." Returning to work after her son's birth, she had scarce time and money. "I don't know if that's a good choice in the long run, but there are two ways I can care for myself and use this time that I have." Ever humorous, she added, "We'll see how it goes. It's a really nice gym."

Hannah, a young woman who had recently graduated from college, made a similar calculation, deciding to spend $100 on 10 yoga classes instead of $100 on a single half-hour therapy session. "That was actually a better solution for me." Phoebe, a value-seeking consumer unwilling to pay $60 per therapy session, made a similar calculation. "I just don't find that as valuable. I would rather pay for a gym membership, to be honest."

Aware of their purchasing role, consumers are positioned to make better—or at least their own—decisions. This is the market at work, where consumers are keenly aware of the value of care and can decide when a service is worth the money.

To therapists, this consumer investment is critical to clinical effectiveness; patients work harder when they pay for the service, and therapy is seen as more effective when consumers work harder at it.

There are obvious downsides of leaving so much to consumers. Psychotherapist Cynthia Reynolds, LCSW, LCAC, remarked that her hairdresser "sets her price based on how many certifications she has, and the level of experience. [But], in our industry, we don't have a way to monitor that because if you only accept cash, you can pretty much do whatever you want. And I think that's really bad for the consumer." There's no way for consumers to assess if someone charging more is better. "There's no governing body that says, 'This person is a level six versus a level two.'" Consumers assess therapists based on convenience or how nice the office is, superficial factors that may not reflect the appropriateness of the care.

IMPROVING ACCESS AND EQUITY IN MENTAL HEALTH

Like dentistry discussed in Chapter 14, mental health care is often separate from the rest of medicine. Inequity between mental health and other health services was prohibited by a 2008 mental health parity law[2] that required organizations offering health benefits to 50 people or more to structure mental health benefits—such as copayments and benefit limits—on par with those for physical health.

Nonetheless, consumers I spoke with were infuriated by lack of access to mental health services.

"The relationship between insurance and mental health is completely flawed and fucked up," Simone told me. A longtime therapy patient whose therapist breakup I described in the Introduction, she scrutinized health insurance options to make sure she and her family would be covered in the event of a crisis, which a family member had previously experienced. "Many plans, the coverage is so flimsy it's shocking. That angers me because it treats mental health as a peripheral issue. I don't think they would do that with cancer treatments. They wouldn't be like, 'Well, you can only have two nights in the hospital.'"

Austin, a graduate student and former nonprofit worker, also expressed anger about disparate mental and physical health coverage. He had opted out of talk therapy, though he felt he would benefit from it because of cost and lack of insurance coverage. "I, for the record, think [that] is criminal. I think that mental health care should be a right for people, but I also think that a smart government invests in the mental health of its people."

Dave, a 50-year-old professional in a technology company, knew about mental health parity rules but felt "the equal standard of care" was not in effect. He paid $160 per session—around $7,000 a year—for his therapy. Initially covered by his employer-sponsored health plan, coverage suddenly stopped when the plan questioned its medical necessity and essentially said he'd been using too much. Dave felt "blacklisted" and cut off from benefits to which he felt entitled. Though he contested the insurance decision, the plan upheld their denial because he appealed too late. He dropped the visit frequency from twice to once a week but continued treatment, paying out of pocket because it improves his productivity and happiness. He wouldn't pay more, though. "The lack of coverage makes me consider very regularly whether to discontinue going."

These consumers reflect broader challenges in access to mental health care. A National Alliance on Mental Illness survey[3] found that respondents were three times more likely to see an out-of-network mental health prescriber,* usually more costly to patients—and four times more likely to see an out-of-network mental health therapist—as they were to see other

---

* "Prescribers" were defined as psychiatrists or other licensed professionals who prescribe medications.

medical specialists out of network. One-third of respondents had trouble finding any mental health therapist or prescriber who would take their insurance, roughly three times more than those reporting trouble finding other in-network medical specialists or primary care providers. About half the mental health professionals were not accepting new patients or insurance at all. Further, respondents reported paying more than $200 out of pocket for these visits almost twice as often as for other specialist visits and primary care visits.[4] Lack of access to psychotherapists who accept insurance often creates financial strain for consumers, putting therapy out of reach for those who simply cannot afford it. And substantial evidence exists of racial and ethnic disparities in access to mental health care.[5]

Parity, it seems, has not yet arrived.

Even without fully enforced parity laws, ample incentive should exist to ensure access to mental health care. Nearly 20% of American adults—43 million people—have some form of mental illness.[6] Mental health and substance use disorders are the leading cause of disease burden and a top-ten cause of death in the United States.[7] Estimates of spending on mental illness range from $110 billion (twice that spent on pregnancy and childbirth)[8] to $240 billion per year,[9] with one study naming mental health disorders the most costly of all categories.[10] Overall treatment—including medical care—for patients with mental illness or substance use disorders cost $752 billion annually.[11] This is not a small category.

Addressing mental health needs would not just be good for patients; it could lower overall health care costs. The average health costs of individuals with mental health or substance use disorders are two to three times those of individuals without such a diagnosis. In addition to direct mental health costs, medical expenses for this group are higher than for people without a mental health or substance use diagnosis.[12] The actuarial firm Milliman estimated that better integration of mental and physical health could save 5% to 10% of overall medical expenses for affected populations, or between $38 and $68 billion per year.[13]

Why, then, isn't mental health coverage more generous?

SHORT SUPPLY

A key feature of the U.S. mental health market is constrained supply of mental health practitioners. Of 28,000 psychiatrists in the United States, three in five are over age 55.[14] Psychiatry training graduates declined by 14% between 2001 and 2008.[15] Despite a modest 5% increase in psychiatry trainees from 2010 to 2015, it will take time to increase the number of practicing psychiatrists.[16] More than 13.5 million adults reported a perceived unmet mental health care need in 2017; 20% of adults with mental illness faced barriers that prevented them from getting the treatment they needed.[17]

One analysis suggested that a shortfall of nearly 6,000 psychiatrists exists.[18] Insufficient supply is measured by the number of federally designated Health Professional Shortage Areas (HPSA) in mental health care. Through September 2019, there were more than 6,000[19] such designations. Nearly 113 million people lived in these shortage areas. Only an estimated 27% of mental health care needs were met.[*,20]

Shrinking supply of mental health care practitioners, as retirements outpace new trainees, is likely to increase demand for remaining psychiatrists. Strong demand allows practitioners to command higher rates and better conditions. In theory, this leverage would extend to negotiating power with insurance companies, but that has not happened. Likely because so many therapists practice on their own or in small groups, individual negotiations tend to favor the health plans, aggregate shortages notwithstanding. As a result, many therapists simply operate outside the insurance system altogether.

The absence of insurance companies as intermediaries is one of the biggest differences between the supply of mental health care services and other types of medicine. A common argument against the feasibility of health care consumerism is the distortion of market signals created by insurers who stand between suppliers and end users. Insurers and providers negotiate rates that employers often pay. Consumers experience the end result, several steps removed from the real pricing and purchasing decisions.

In mental health care, though, for better and worse, there is less noise and clearer signal between providers and consumers. Just as consumers are customers, providers are sellers. In that role, providers more directly serve consumers and practice according to their own preferences and tolerances.

INSURANCE DISINCENTIVES

"It is like having a dictator from outside the room, orchestrating your treatments, which to me is orchestrating a relationship. That just doesn't

---

* The Henry J. Kaiser Family Foundation calculates the percentage of needs met by dividing the number of psychiatrists available to serve the population of the area, group, or facility by the number of psychiatrists that would be necessary to eliminate the mental health HPSA (based on a ratio of 30,000 to 1 or 20,000 to 1 where high needs are indicated). *Source*: https://www.kff.org/other/state-indicator/mental-health-care-health-professional-shortage-areas-hpsas/.

seem like good medicine to me," Beth Nierenberg described the impact of health insurers on clinical care. A seasoned licensed mental health counselor in private practice, Nierenberg objects to the sometimes-heavy-handed requirements and criteria insurance companies impose on clinicians. "I very specifically decided no one was going to tell me how to do my job. I wasn't going to give people 200-question assessments on the hello and diagnose them before the second session. That's outside my belief system and what's good for people and why people engage in treatment."

I also spoke with a psychologist who specializes in neuropsychological testing and therapy for children; I'll call her Dr. Z.* Dr. Z most often sees patients outside insurance, "to have more control over number of sessions and all of that," she told me. "I find it is certainly very disruptive to be making progress and having to stop because insurance is not covering things." Insurance companies tend to be rigid about benefit approvals, when clinicians need and want flexibility in treating individual patients.

A highly specialized psychiatrist practicing privately in New York City—I'll call him Dr. A—said other than when he was employed by institutions, "I don't think I've ever in my life taken a check from an insurance company, nor would I want to." He, too, objected to clinical interference. "It's intrusive in the doctor-patient relationship," he said. The insurance company "can dictate how long you can meet for, how much you can meet, what the parameters of treatment are. It's bad enough they dictate pharmacology. I find it offensive." He tells patients his decision not to accept insurance means that "you and I get to decide how long we'll meet for, not a third party."

Cynthia Reynolds practices both in private practice—where she addresses costs directly—and in a clinic, where it is someone else's job to manage billing. She appreciates the help: "It allows me to really focus on patient care."

THE ALMIGHTY DOLLAR

In addition to the clinical autonomy refusing insurance provides, there are very real financial considerations for private-practice mental health clinicians.

"Insurance fees tend to be low and you have to fight to get them." Dr. A told me. "They can arbitrarily carve out visits because they decide that it wasn't medically necessary." Ironically, in this way, insurers demonstrate

---

* I spoke with several psychiatrists and psychologists about their practices and offered them anonymity because of the proprietary details they shared with me.

less willingness than therapists to participate in the market. Insurance reimbursement rates are often set centrally, without effective responsiveness to market conditions. Unmet demand from supply shortages could be remedied, at least in part, with higher insurance reimbursements. But such remedies would cost insurers more, a clear disincentive for change. Moreover, some economists caution that precisely because people are willing to pay out of pocket for mental health services, more generous insurance coverage is unnecessary and could lead to over-utilization.[21] This argument rests heavily on the flawed assumption that mental health care is less likely to be medically necessary than other medical services.

"Imagine if you went to a restaurant, sat down, ordered a meal," Dr. A set up a hypothetical scenario. "A waiter gave you the check and it was for 100 bucks. And you said, 'I'll give you $65.'" Presumably, the waiter would say, "We don't barter here." Or he might ask, "Why? Was there a problem with the service?" Dr. A sees himself as the waiter—or the restaurant—and the insurance company is the diner, arbitrarily deciding what to pay as if the restaurant has no role in setting its own price. In that system, only the insurer can negotiate. The restaurant can take $65 or nothing at all.

No matter what someone charges, insurance pays so much less; it caused Beth Nierenberg to consider the downsides of accepting insurance on her well-being as well as her bank account. "I have to see four times as many people to make the same amount of money."

Another psychologist in a group practice he built over several years—I'll call him Dr. Y—used round numbers to illustrate this point. "If I have an open spot and I can fill that spot with somebody using their insurance, I'll get paid 100 bucks. Or I can fill that spot with somebody that I'm going to see that will pay $200. I will feel better seeing the person for $200, if all other factors are equal. I want to try to protect the patient against me agreeing to a situation that I'm not going to feel good about."

"Your compensation is really much lower than in private practice," Dr. Z agreed, describing the financial equation of accepting insurance. "For therapy, you might get reimbursed about three-quarters of your fee, whereas for [neuropsychology], it's about half." Insurers offer less reimbursement for the service in shorter supply, at least as a percentage of her charges, presumably because the fees are higher and many consumers, themselves, are willing to pay. Given Dr. Z's specialization, families often reach her via referral, desperate to be seen. They're usually educated about what they need, aware of the general costs and that insurance won't pay, and not particularly price sensitive. "I rarely have anyone push back," she said. "I don't think I charge as much as I could."

Even when clinicians are willing to accept insurance, administrative hassles create other costs. Whenever Dr. Z has tried to get insurance reimbursement, she winds up getting "into fights with insurance companies that end up taking a long amount of time, not getting paid, and having to go back to the family anyway." Instead, she prepares an invoice for patients who want to try to get insurance reimbursement on their own, though she hesitates to unduly raise patient expectations. She discloses up front that "I'm not going to get involved in negotiating with their insurance company." Even if she could accept the decreased reimbursement, it's just not worth the time and headache involved.

It might be tempting to chalk these sentiments up to greed, but psychiatrists are among the least well compensated of all physician specialties, coming in 19th out of 29 specialties in a 2017 compensation survey, earning about half what the top earners brought in.[22]

PROVIDERS AS SELLERS

Without insurance stipulating rules and rates, providers are free to set their own terms. The psychiatrists and psychologists I interviewed were thoughtful and intentional about the business of mental health. Their rate-setting approaches were largely market driven, like any other service provider.

"I do ask around to see what other people charge, and I would say I am probably in the middle of my colleagues who do private practice," Dr. Z told me. She is occasionally surprised to hear what others are charging when she comes across colleagues' fees, but she, herself, does not try to maximize her earnings. "I'm too much of a softie," she joked. Though she avoids insurance, she uses insurance reimbursement as a benchmark setting her own fees, knowing that private practice commands higher rates.

Dr. Y admitted, "It's very unscientific." He compares what he understands peers to be charging and pegs his rate in the middle. "My most grandiose and narcissistic peers are significantly higher. My most self-effacing and neurotically self-denigrating peers are less. And I want to be somewhere between those two." His rate is wrapped up in his own sense of self. "My practice reflects my class identity. There are middle-class clinicians who have nobody paying their full fee . . . and there are genuinely upper-middle-class clinicians who only see people who pay their full fee. I'm sort of lower-upper-middle class."

Dr. Y also factors "supply and demand." He tries to feel the pulse of his patient population. "It's some intuitive calculation about the people who can afford to pay out of pocket" and what they're willing to pay. After a long time, he raised his rate, realizing the difference would likely be more noticeable to him in a positive way than to his patients in a negative way. And patients have been willing to pay. Less-experienced clinicians in his practice charge a lower rate. "Their patients probably couldn't go that much higher," he explained. "I'd rather have my clinicians seeing people for $140 than not seeing people at all." It's also better than the $100 they might get in insurance reimbursement.

Cynthia Reynolds also knows she could charge more but works at keeping her rate accessible. "I'm very well aware that there are therapists with less experience who were charging 50% more than what I charge. I would like my cash price to be reasonable so that people can afford it and so that they can see me consistently."

Dr. A sets his private-pay rate carefully so as not to violate antitrust laws. "You get a sense, informally, of what's the usual and customary," and he tries to fall within that range. He provides a premium service, almost concierge style, in exchange. "Patients who complain they can never reach their other doctors, you'll hear back from me pretty quick, but that comes at a cost. So, I'd say I'm charging what I think most senior New York City-area psychiatrists charge and maybe the same or a little less than some of the hoity-toity, big-shot luminaries out there."

Dr. B, another psychologist in private practice, similarly does not seek to maximize his earnings. "It's partly my own countertransference," he laughed, using a psychoanalytic term for his feelings about his patients. "But I'm 64, right? I'm probably not going to change." He explained, "I tend to take a little more responsibility than I should fee-wise for the patients feeling comfortable. I don't want the financial ties to intrude on it." He acknowledges his approach may be naive, "But, I like being fair, more than fair. It gets me comfortable in the room." Most of the time, he feels he is delivering value to patients and senses his patients get a lot out of his services. "But every once in a while you think, 'This is a weird service to be providing,'" he laughed. "Should they be paying for this?" Those moments are few and far between for this seasoned clinician, but knowing he has offered a more-than-fair financial deal helps him move through those moments more easily.

When Beth Nierenberg set her private-practice rates after working for many years in human services agencies serving "people living absolutely at the edges of poverty," she felt awkward. "The idea of charging someone in a way that was going to cause them to write a check felt impossible to me." She learned to focus on the value she brought to patients and to trust that people are willing to pay for that value.

THE POWER OF PRICE TRANSPARENCY

Though many consumers can tell horror stories about surprise medical bills and fights with health insurers, surprise bills are exceedingly rare in mental health. "Do you ever get a surprise bill?" I asked dozens of consumers who discussed psychotherapy. "Of course not!" they would chide me. Their therapists had proactively discussed the fees up front, before the first visit.

"Usually I find they tell you on the phone before you go," Simone said. Paulette described this pre-visit process. "I knew going in. She told me up front. She said, 'I don't take insurance. This is what it is.'" Paulette made an informed decision about an expensive service.

Therapists confirmed that price disclosure is no mistake. Unlike medical providers who often do not know or discuss prices with patients, therapists consistently put costs on the table explicitly. Psychotherapists were clear: financial hardship does not make for a healthy therapeutic relationship for anyone involved. To avoid such challenges, they learn on the job to discuss costs up front and if someone's financial situation changes in the midst of treatment.

"I don't like sticker shock any more than they do," Dr. A explained his screening process to make sure he is an appropriate therapist for prospective patients who call for appointments. "Up front, I typically will say to patients, 'Just so you're aware, I have a specialty practice. I'm not in network with any insurance plan. My fee is expensive.'" If someone expresses concern about the cost, Dr. A typically refers them to other clinicians who might charge lower rates or accept insurance. "Health care should never be a hardship."

Dr. A emphasized he is also screening for fit, an important feature of effective therapeutic relationships. "It's a little bit like that TV show 'The Voice,' where your chair swings around and you're listening to what the person has to say. And you're trying to decide if you think you can work with them, and if you want to work with them. And if you're not sure, don't turn your chair around. It's kind of a vetting process or filtering process. Do I think I have something that can help you?" Fees may be just one ingredient in that determination; the therapists I interviewed care a lot about delivering value.

Beth Nierenberg also vets new patients and wants them to vet her. "I tell them exactly what I cost. I tell them I don't take insurance. I let them know that I'm happy to meet with them first for free." She encourages patients to assess, "Am I even the right kind of person for you?" Sometimes people call knowing they want to work with her, while others come through layers of referrals. "Those people, I would like to meet them. I would like them to meet me. I would like to have a better understanding of what they're looking for in terms of focus and skill set because I am not the only game in town. There [are] 100 therapists within ten feet of the door of my office." This sounds like a market wherein supply and demand are closely aligned. If Nierenberg were a classic merchant, she'd be the type who encouraged prospective purchasers to "try before they buy."

As in clinical autonomy and total compensation, insurance involvement for those who accept it foils price disclosures because no one knows what, if anything, insurance will reimburse. "You can't always pin it down," Dr. B said.

Some of Dr. Y's patients seek insurance reimbursement, but he can't tell them what to expect ahead of time. Reimbursement might be 70% or 80% of "usual, customary, and reasonable" charges, a standard rate determined to be the norm for a given service. Reimbursement is not based on what the therapist charges but rather on what the health plan deems standard. "They won't tell you what that rate is ahead of time. So, the only way to know what insurance will actually pay out is to submit claims." Insurance makes it hard for therapists to be transparent.

COST-CONVERSATION COMPETENCY

Price transparency in therapy is possible in part because therapists overcome early career discomfort to develop a competency in discussing money.

"They don't teach you in grad school how to talk to somebody about what you charge," Beth Nierenberg explained. "They don't tell you how to set a fee. They don't tell you how to decide whether you're going to take insurance. . . . Some of that, you have to figure out on your own."

Dr. B explained why these conversations can be so hard. "I think it's this idea that you're a caregiver in a sensitive area of health and that it's somehow wrong to put that before the well-being of a patient in your office." Therapists with less experience sometimes assume "that most patients are more vulnerable than they are to discussions in general" and discount patients' ability to talk about sensitive topics without falling apart or harshly judging the clinician. "I've come to appreciate that it's just better for them, too, to have it be clear in the beginning."

Cynthia Reynolds is also conscientious about these conversations. "When someone contacts me as a new patient, I have to find out what is bringing them to therapy while also finding out what they can afford either through their insurance or through cash before going much further." Raising cost as the first topic feels inconsiderate but she has learned the hard way not to wait too long. "I've made all kinds of mistakes, going so far as scheduling the person and then at the very last part of the conversation, bringing up cost, finding out that that doesn't fit into their budget, and then canceling the appointment." Now, she assesses if she can help the patient *and* if they are comfortable with her fees. She discloses her cash price and the negotiated rate she has to charge if the patient uses his or her insurance, recognizing that people on high-deductible plans pay that rate directly, particularly early in the year.

Reynolds is also conscientious about collecting payments. "If a person that wants to come in and perhaps not come back or not pay their bill, I think what they're doing is they're taking away perhaps from somebody that wants to come in." To keep her fees accessible even to people with very high deductibles, she explained, "I need to make sure, like any business, that I am collecting appropriate fees."

Dr. B also learned the hard way to have cost conversations. "Early on, I had more difficulty approaching it," he said. "I actually got burned a couple of times because of that. And now, I'm very flexible in what I arrange with patients, but it's clear." He tries to engage in direct conversations about cost. "Most of the time, it's a very straightforward conversation," he said. "I think clear expectations are better."

Dr. B added, "There's enough weird stuff in therapy. . . . It's part of my style to have straightforward things be straightforward, and finances get included in that." Depending on the patient, he might approach the conversation more delicately. "I just want them to be okay and reassure them that if for some reason it's not making sense to them, the financial arrangements, that I'm there or I'll be there until they have a more solid [arrangement] with someone else."

Cost conversations are about more than money. Naming one's fee involves declaring one's worth, about which therapists can feel sheepish, especially at first.

Dr. Y explained, "As I am more confident in the value of my skills for people and that I'm really giving them something that will be transformative in their lives, I feel more comfortable talking with them about the money because I think they will get something really worthwhile." He emphasized the importance of up-front cost conversations in part as a way of seeking certainty that he can add value.

These conversations may not feel natural at first, but therapists learn to overcome their own insecurities, discomfort, and concern for patients. Therapists demonstrate both the ability to and the importance of engaging with patients on financial matters; they develop systems and approaches to doing so. They learn from these encounters and evolve.

PCPs and clinicians in other specialties deal with more complexity, more billing codes, and more insurance involvement. Nonetheless, they could and should follow therapists' example. Like it or not, concerted efforts to train medical students about costs—although relatively new and not necessarily effective yet[23]—likely portend a future in which doctors look more like therapists in terms of discussing costs openly.

NEGOTIATING

Flowing from initial cost disclosure, and the relative lack of insurance involvement, therapists have flexibility to negotiate rates. Their willingness to negotiate depends on factors like how busy they are when someone asks for a price break, how established they are, and how confident they are in the value of their services.

Busy clinicians are less willing to negotiate with new patients. Dr. Y, established in his career, rarely slides his fee to fill his schedule. "If people call, I want to be helpful. It's very hard for me emotionally to say 'no' just because of money. But at this point, if people have a significant problem with my fee, I just give them other options."

To maintain long-term, positive relationships, though, "I generally try not to let money interfere with relations," Dr. Y said. "I'll slide significantly for somebody I'm in an established treatment with whose circumstances have changed." Dr. A is similarly more flexible with current patients. "They achieve a certain elite status. If I think I'm helpful to them and if my experience with them is a positive one, I have flexibility." Dr. A sometimes even offers to treat people for less if he knows they're struggling and that he's helping. "I want to do good work."

Dr. Y is more willing to negotiate "if it's somebody that I really want to work with." That desire to work with someone might be to maintain a good relationship with whomever referred them, if the patient needs to feel like he or she is getting a small price break but it's not a steep discount, or if someone is clinically compelling. Most importantly, this willingness to work with patients on price comes down to feeling like the patient is benefiting from the relationship.

Dr. B confirmed "how much I would like to see the patient" is an important factor in whether he slides his fee. "There's a whole gestalt; who are they? How much [do] they need to come? How often did I see them? Are they people of means? Are they nice to work with? There will be a whole sort of gestalt of factors that go into when there's a shift like that."

One of Beth Nierenberg's specialties is gender nonconforming children, sometimes with medical issues. "When that kid shows up in my office, I'm not quick to refer out." Sometimes, a close colleague refers patients to her, saying, "You're their person. They need you." When she knows she has the right experience to serve their specific "cluster of needs," she hates to turn them away. She'll work with families to figure out what benefits they might be able to access and how she can help make the finances work.

The decision to negotiate involves more than pure financial considerations. It is also about setting limits and learning how patients respond to challenging situations. It's also about how the therapist feels.

"You don't want to set up a situation in which you have any negative feelings about seeing the person because then you can't be helpful," Dr. Y coaches the clinicians who work for him. "If you agree to a situation that you're going to end up resenting, it's not going to be in the patient's best interest."

Dr. B has adjusted to the financial dimension of therapy. "I'm totally comfortable in the fact that this is how I make my living, and I don't apologize for that. But I also want to be sure it's a comfortable match because

I don't want to negotiate down my fee to where I feel bad about it and I don't want them to be over-paying because they'll feel bad about it. I almost feel like that's an obstacle to success on either side, and therefore, better not to start in those situations."

Underpinning all these therapists' willingness to slide their fees more for certain patients than others is that therapists derive satisfaction from treating patients whom they feel genuinely benefit from their services. That satisfaction turns out to be worth money to them. Therapists want to treat people they can help. The therapeutic alliance, described in Chapter 9 as a measure and predictor of quality, seems as important to therapists as it is to patients.

HOW CONSUMERS CAN TRY NEGOTIATING THERAPY FEES

Patients who feel they need therapy but who struggle with the cost may try these negotiating approaches:

1. Offer to pay up front if that's not already part of the arrangement.
2. Pay with cash or check—it costs the therapist less than processing a credit card.
3. Leave a credit card on file to protect the therapist from you not paying.
4. Be flexible with your scheduling; see if there's a day or time that would be helpful for the therapist to fill.
5. Commit to your therapeutic relationship; the more you benefit from therapy, the more invested your therapist will likely be. Of course, you can't fake that. Your therapist will know.

THE THERAPY MODEL

Ironically, the part of the U.S. health care system that is often cited as reflecting dysfunction may serve as a model of consumerism. Psychotherapy positions consumers squarely as purchasers, for better and worse, because so much of it takes place outside of insurance rules. As a result of paying out of pocket, consumers know their role and calculate the value of therapy to them. They shop around and seek therapists who fit their needs and their wallets. They know what therapy costs before the service occurs and pay at the point of purchase. Balances rarely accrue. When rates become burdensome, therapists often flex to maintain long-term therapeutic relationships. Payment options, themselves, can be flexible and convenient.

Psychotherapy provides an opportunity to observe market forces—however imperfect—at work in health care. Therapists and patients interact transactionally even as they build deep clinical relationships. Pricing and billing are simpler, in large part because of the relatively small set of services available but also because of choices therapists make to establish prices, disclose them, and set clear expectations up front. Consumers know exactly what therapy is worth to them. If they question the value, they can negotiate or stop going.

Providers, on the other hand, acknowledge that they earn their living from patient fees. They grow into levels of comfort with the act of charging money for their time, as they gain experience and confidence in the value they deliver to patients. They calculate what they can afford to negotiate, both financially and emotionally.

If the broader health care system resembled the best of mental health care, it would set clear and rational fees, based on the value of providers' time and service. Clinicians would have clinical autonomy, not unduly encumbered by insurance rules. And they would set their own prices and stand by them, facing the consumer directly. Open, authentic, proactive communication about cost would be the norm. Payment would be efficient, convenient, and timely. Huge bills would not accrue, creating administrative and financial burdens for consumers and providers alike. There would be less need for giant billing departments and for consumers to go into collections or providers to write off massive amounts of uncollected debt. And consumers would know their place: in control of their choices and entitled to care that works for them.

4

Shopper, Know Thyself

How different types of people engage with health care differently

"We did market research," said the woman at the front of the Brown University classroom. "And we found that some people don't *like* raisins in their granola." She was there on behalf of her advertising agency, recruiting summer interns from my undergraduate class. At the time, I had no plans or prospects for the summer.

Had I been drinking something, I would have spit it out, sitcom style, unable to contain myself. "You had to do MARKET RESEARCH to know that?" my inner voice screamed, incredulous yet somehow managing to keep quiet. "I could have told you that for free!" Not only did I not apply for that internship, but I also wrote off the whole advertising industry as idiotic.

Decades later, I stand corrected. After discovering a love of consumer marketing and spending my career in the field, I have countless market research projects and advertising campaigns under my belt. I have a more nuanced appreciation of advertising and understand the power of marketing to discover and connect to consumer needs and desires.

Moreover, I now think the raisins-in-granola woman could be helpful in health care, where millions of Americans pay approximately one-third[1,2] of expenses out of pocket yet are scarcely recognized as consumers. The same people who distinguished granola-with-raisin lovers from haters could shed light on the many different types of health care purchasers, just as they have segmented consumers in other consumer markets.

Segmentation is the basic process of dividing things—or people—into separate groups. In marketing terms, this process involves dividing the world of potential customers based on shared characteristics. The ad agency that first exposed me to this concept had divided granola eaters into pro-raisin people and anti-raisiners. Commonly, segmentation divides along concrete demographic lines, like age, gender, geography, or income. These divisions make it relatively easy to reach the target segment, such as with billboards targeting a specific neighborhood or TV ads during a certain time of day. If you ever flip on middle-of-the-night TV, I promise you will see ads for sleep aids and probably drug and alcohol rehabilitation facilities. These ads tell you who else is watching when you are.

Other bases for segmentation group people according to how they buy things: price-sensitive shoppers versus brand-conscious ones, impulse buyers, or research-driven purchasers. Some retailers have multiple brands to reach these different shoppers. Banana Republic-Gap-Old Navy are owned by the same company but target different consumer segments. Most car companies have a plethora of brands and models to allow them to reach different kinds of car buyers. Large consumer-packaged goods companies manage families of individual brands, often aimed at different parts of the same markets. Sometimes the segments are so different that the companies try to hide their other affiliations. I remember one of my business school classmate's horrified disillusionment when he learned that his brawny DeWalt tools were manufactured by Black and Decker, maker of delightfully convenient small home appliances.

My favorite segmentation schemes are along psychographic dimensions—those inner traits and characteristics that explain what makes people tick. Are you an Info Seeker, a News Junkie, or a Deal Seeker[3] in your media consumption habits? When you travel, are you the Collector, the Conformist, the Thrill-Seeker, or the Escapist?[4] The cooler and more evocative the label, the better.

In health care, segmenting providers is common. Providers are logically grouped by training (such as MDs vs. RNs), by specialty (cardiology vs. dermatology), by practice setting (hospital or clinic based), or by insurance status (in or out of network). Whole organizations exist to convene and represent individual provider specialties. A health care venture capitalist I spoke to likened these associations to trade unions, because they so powerfully protect the interests of their members.

Consumer segmentation in health care is increasingly recognized as important, but in practical application, it still largely focuses on disease states and service utilization. Health plans maintain registries—or databases—of diabetic members, asthmatics, and cancer patients and deploy nurses or social workers to help those members manage their care.

A huge amount of health industry focus is on "high utilizers" or "frequent fliers"—the 5% to 10% of any group who use the most services and therefore cost the most. Analyses of high-cost members divide people with complex health care needs by how much money they cost the health plan each month or year. Entrepreneurs and investors are flocking to these high-cost, complex segments, where introducing even small efficiencies can yield oversized financial returns.

Looking at health care consumers in terms of how much they cost the system—instead of how they spend their health care dollars—takes consumers out of the equation or at least out of the center of it. This mentality hones in on the greatest leverage points for addressing health care costs—the most costly patients—but also lumps together people on measures that may not reflect much about how they make health care decisions, what they care about, or what motivates them. Thus, it does not offer any mechanism to influence or engage with health care consumers on a deeper level.

"To study a lower-order characteristic of the consumer is to take a narrow view of the market," wrote Seymour Fine, a social marketing expert and marketing professor at Rutgers University until 2002, in a 1980 paper.[5] His concept was to segment consumers according to their objectives rather than simply on their consumption patterns. Though consumer marketing and segmentation has evolved significantly since 1980—and Professor Fine, himself, kept writing on marketing for years after that early work—Fine's main point still applies to health care consumer segmentation. Consumers' goals for themselves influence their consumption decisions and therefore can provide a richer, more nuanced basis for segmenting consumers.

Today, many health care consumer segmentation schemes exist. Deloitte, a global accounting and consulting firm, identified six health care consumer segments based on attitudes and behaviors. These segments, derived from and validated with thousands of consumer surveys, include categories like "casual and cautious," "content and compliant," and "online and onboard."[6] One market research firm, cb2, divides health care consumers along psychographic measures into five segments, including "self-achiever," "direction taker," and "willful endurer."[7] Their model, also based on surveys with thousands of consumers, describes groups with different attitudes and priorities and proposes different communication approaches depending on the segment. Altarum, a nonprofit health care research and consulting firm, developed and validated the ACE measure, its own measure of health care consumer engagement,[8] based on different consumer profiles.

All such segmentation approaches are designed to help health care organizations better understand and reach, sell to, or design programs for different types of health care consumers. Whether someone extensively researches their prospective doctor's credentials and ratings before making an appointment or can't be bothered to go to the doctor at all has practical implications for health systems and insurers. If companies can figure out who's who and offer the right information, tools, and messages to the right segments, that starts to sound like progress toward a higher-functioning consumer market.

TRANSCENDING POLITICS IN HEALTH CARE SHOPPING

I had the opportunity to collaborate with RealClear Politics and their Opinion Research arm on a poll they conducted about American voters' attitudes toward health care in the spring of 2019. The survey of 2,000 voters[9] showed that 62% of respondents felt health care was one of the two most important issues facing the United States, and nearly three-quarters of respondents felt the U.S. health system is broken or not working well.

The survey allowed my research collaborators and me to identify meaningful health care consumer segments[10] and understand how those consumer segments might relate to voting patterns and political persuasions. Using a clustering algorithm, we found four distinct groups within the broader poll and examined what characteristics other than their responses to survey questions distinguished the groups from one another. After looking at a wide range of demographic factors like age, education, and political affiliation, we found the segments divided along two main dimensions: (1) satisfaction with health care and (2) propensity to shop in a health care context (or actively engage with their health care decisions).[11]

What kind of health care consumer someone was, in this analysis, had more to do with age, education, and overall outlook than with political ideology or party affiliation. Each segment had a unique profile:

1. Satisfied and savvy

Nearly a quarter (24%) of Americans in the survey were contented and capable health care shoppers. They were generally satisfied with the quality and value of their health care. Whether cause or effect, they tended to report higher levels of engagement with their decisions than other segments. They reported paying close attention to health costs, comparing options, checking health care prices ahead of time, and researching doctors online. Though least likely to cite lowering health care costs as their top priority, almost half reported feeling burdened by their own health care costs.

Optimistic—likely because of their own good health care experiences—they were most likely to assume others get good health care. This group was the most educated and wealthy of the segments, the most politically engaged segment, and more likely to have a party affiliation. They were open to health reform proposals and valued health insurance portability. Competent in navigating the current system, they were also open minded about proposed health reforms.

2. Skeptical and searching

Active and cost-conscious shoppers, this group represented one-fifth (19%) of the survey population. These consumers were highly engaged in health care decisions, researching options and closely monitoring their health costs. However, they were not happy with their health care. The majority (68%) felt burdened by health costs, more than any other segment. They were most likely to care about ensuring all Americans get access to health care, probably because they, themselves, feel vulnerable. They did not assume others have great health care (21%) because their own care was not satisfying to them. Demographically, this group had the largest percentage of Millennials and the smallest proportion of older Americans. They were least likely to be high-income earners and most likely to identify as Independent voters who felt the country is on the wrong track. This group tended to support health reform proposals that eliminate private insurers.

3. Unhappy and unplugged

Consumers in this segment—representing 25% of the population—were both dissatisfied and unengaged with their health care. They weren't prone to shop around or research their options. This group cared more than others did about access to substance use disorder services and less about making sure everyone can access care. A quarter of them prioritized price transparency as a most pressing issue in health care, more than other segments. They were less educated and had lower income than other groups. They were the least politically engaged group, with almost one-fifth sitting out the 2016 presidential election. Though they reported the highest opposition of any group to Medicare for All proposals, their support improved when presented as a path to eliminating private insurers. It is safe to say this group is relatively "anti-establishment," as it has not felt well served by the status quo.

4. Coasting and contented

These consumers—nearly a third of respondents (31%)—were satisfied non-shoppers. They did not shop or engage in health care decisions as much as other segments. They were least likely to feel burdened by health care costs (34%), fully half as much as the most burdened group. They cared a lot about lowering the cost of prescription drugs (44%) and making sure doctors—not insurers—make health care decisions (41%). They focused more than others did on protections for people with preexisting conditions (42%) and were less concerned about cost transparency (18%). This was the oldest group, with the fewest young adults. They were least supportive of health reform proposals that eliminate private health insurance compared to other groups. Based on the age distribution, this group is likely over-representative of Medicare enrollees, who are known to be happier than most, on average, with their health care.[12] In Chapter 15, I take a closer look at Medicare and its enrollees.

These segments start to give shape to different types of health care shoppers and how politicians courting health care voters may want to target their policy proposals and health care messaging.

WHAT KIND OF SHOPPER ARE *YOU*?

In a less-scientific exercise, over the course of more than 60 consumer interviews about people's experiences with and feelings about health care purchasing, I began to recognize distinct health care shopping types or personalities. The most meaningful dimensions I observed were degrees of financial motivation, levels of trust or lack thereof, and orientation toward activity or passivity. Based on these observations, I have identified 12 different types of health care shoppers. Each type appears to respond differently to health care information, base their health care purchase decisions on different criteria, and conceptualize their role in health care purchasing differently.

These shopper types are not necessarily fixed. That is, people may behave as one type in certain situations and a different type in other contexts. Though these personae are not derived analytically or quantitatively validated, they illustrate important differences among health care consumers and illuminate key dimensions along which these differences fall.

Let me introduce you to some of the representative characters I met, in no particular order. Do you recognize yourself in any of these descriptions?

The Organizer

When Margaret found herself stuck between her health plan and her therapist in a billing snafu, she organized her records and traced her past visits, bills already paid, and outstanding balances. She sorted out who should pay what portion of the outstanding balances. In Chapter 7, I describe her story more fully. Margaret recognized the onus is on the patient to navigate. "You have to be educated and pay attention to it, it being the way the health care system works and insurance, and reading the details and advocating for yourself, so that you get the right care at the right cost or whatever the cost is supposed to be." She doesn't love that reality, but she manages it. "It felt more complicated than it needs to be, but that is the system."

Are You an Organizer?

Organizers operate as efficiently as possible within the current health system—messy and broken though it is. They would fare relatively well in any system because they rely on themselves to navigate. They keep track of costs and the services they need or have used. They independently assess the value of services and the fairness of the charges. They're rational, tidy, and clear in their thinking. They are driven by order and fairness more than by money itself. Their dominant feature appears to be organization, but, at the core, their most important traits are confidence, competence, and self-reliance.

The Negotiator

Ralph—who features in Chapters 6 and 9—loves to negotiate so much that friends and family call on him to get them the best possible price on their new cars. "If I can negotiate something, I'll try to negotiate it," he told me. He negotiated with a doctor after insurance rejected part of a claim, and the balance—which he felt he shouldn't have to pay—fell to Ralph. When he could not get the doctor to budge on the price, Ralph let the doctor know not to count on him for a positive reference. But Ralph remained undeterred from trying to negotiate in the future. He's always willing to try.

Are You a Negotiator?

Negotiators enjoy bartering. For them, negotiating is like sport. They generally care more about getting a better deal than about the absolute price. Sometimes they negotiate just to see what they can get. They confront costs head on. They are not shy or sensitive about asking. They are curious about what they can get from their negotiations. They do not feel insecure about what negotiating may signal about them. They have confidence and the energy to hold providers accountable for delivering fair value. They would rather win, but they're more afraid of not trying—and potentially leaving money on the table—than of failing.

The Value Seeker

Phoebe, a young professional, decided to get Invisalign to straighten her teeth before leaving a high-paying corporate job where she had good health benefits. Her flexible spending account would expire soon, and she shopped around to compare prices to stretch her savings as far as possible. "This will be the cheapest it probably will ever be for me," she said. Adam took value-seeking to a whole other level when he helped the small company he worked for choose health insurance. With a new baby on the way, Adam was the only one of his young colleagues who anticipated any near-term substantial health expenses. He realized he could cover the difference in premium for his colleagues and still save money on a lower-deductible plan. The lengths these two were willing to go in order to maximize economic value appear in Chapter 13.

Are You a Value Seeker?

Value Seekers are the most cost-conscious health care consumers, no matter how much money they actually have. They nose out the most efficient path to value. Whether motivated by financial hardship or just a quest for the best deal, they are incentive driven and make health care decisions based explicitly on cost. If there is a cheaper way to get what they need, they will find it. If not, they might avoid care until their health need becomes urgent.

The Sheriff

Rosemary strenuously argued with her insurance company on several occasions for coverage she felt they should provide, as described in Chapters 5, 8, and 13. Though the money was an important factor for her—she did not want to pay more than she had to—the driving force for her was fairness and the right answer. In one instance, Rosemary found herself caught in a catch-22 situation for her daughter's medication. The medications on the health plan's preferred drug list weren't dosed for a peanut-sized toddler; the only drug she could take cost $30 more per prescription than a preferred drug would. "It's not my fault she can't take one of the preferred drugs because she's only 27 pounds!" Rosemary took the case as far as she could, without success. Her own ability to pay the full fee was of limited comfort. "What if this was a medication that she needed to survive and we could not afford it?" This concern for justice and care for others moves Rosemary beyond an expert self-advocator. It makes her a Sheriff.

Are You a Sheriff?

Sheriffs know the rules—or think they do—and do their best to hold people accountable to them. They will fight bills and appeal decisions they feel are unfair or incorrect. They value the savings they may achieve, but it is more important to them to fight on principle. As a result, they will pursue this version of justice to the end of the road, no matter how frustrating or time consuming.

The Accepter

Theo appears in Chapters 3 and 5. He is clear that the time he would spend seeking corrections or accommodation to bills that do not seem right would likely only yield frustration for him. Whatever money he might get back is not worth his aggravation. "I'm not a negotiator," Theo said. "I don't call someone to save $50. But that's my life. I'm endlessly feeling taken advantage of by the system and just resigned to it. . . . I have, on occasion, called about things like this, but it never works out."

Are You an Accepter?

Accepters are health care consumers who recognize how complex and broken American health care is and that they cannot fix it. The game is rigged against them, and there is little point in trying to fight it. The aggravation involved is not worth the value they could get if they fight. They preserve their energy for other pursuits, and engage with the health system only when they must. If getting their due seems like it will require energy, it's not worth it. Admit defeat. Cut losses. Move on.

The Trusting Soul

Hazel has a sunny disposition. Living in a resort town with her husband, two kids, and her own business, she feels like every day is her birthday. In Chapter 12, I share her story, and explain how she never considered shopping for her own health insurance. Instead, Hazel found an agent and went with her recommendation. "I trust people to do what they know," she told me. Because health insurance is confusing, she assumes the people who deal in it every day are best equipped to advise her. As a graphic design professional with her own expertise, she is accustomed to people seeking her services without really knowing what they need and trusting her to figure out and deliver the best solutions. She trusts others will do the same for her. Despite her optimism, she told me, "I feel pretty certain that mistakes have been made and I've paid more than I should at different times. It wouldn't be reasonable to expect otherwise, but it's one of those things that stinks, but it feels a little bit out of my hands." There are only so many hours in a day, and fighting with her insurance company or second guessing her medical bills is not how she wants to spend her precious time.

Are You a Trusting Soul?

Trusting Souls are the shiny side of the Accepters' coin. Where Accepters are sure they are getting screwed, Trusting Souls recognize that possibility but don't let it get them down. Like Accepters, they understand that health care doesn't always work that well, but they assume it generally works well enough. And life is short. Go smell some flowers!

The Spender

"There isn't a price tag," Sabrina said of her daughter's health. In Chapter 9, I share her story of facing a delicate endocrinology treatment decision relating to her young daughter. Though Sabrina argued with her insurance plan to cover the out-of-network consultation, it didn't matter much to her that she was unsuccessful. It's not that she earns so much money; in fact, she says she lives paycheck to paycheck. But she has savings to draw from and values good medical advice as well as her time. "There was never a question in my mind that I wasn't going to get a second opinion."

Are You a Spender?

Spenders have a level of financial security that allows them to focus on getting the best care from the best providers. They are not necessarily wealthy or spoiled, though they have enough resources to prioritize their health or their family's health. Unlike Value Seekers, Spenders are willing to pay for the confidence that they're in the right hands. They may tend to choose the health insurance that gives them the maximum flexibility—the widest selection of doctors and hospitals, with the least amount of bureaucratic hassle to see who they want to see when they want to see them. They are not, and likely never will be, price sensitive. They're least likely to ask what things cost, and there's no chance they'd ever negotiate or shop around—unless there might be better-quality option available.

The Aspiring Shopper

"I would want more options," Brooke reflected on her experience buying individual insurance on the health insurance marketplace created by the Affordable Care Act. She represents a new generation of health care shoppers, and I share more of her sentiments in Chapter 12. Brooke isn't accustomed to such limiting shopping experiences. Having come of age in the digital era, she expects a wide array of options, including ones that suit her needs. She didn't find those on the insurance marketplace, and she couldn't understand why not. "I feel like that would probably drive cost down, if there's more to choose from and more competition."

Are You an Aspiring Shopper?

Some people don't understand why health care is so different from everything else they spend their money on. Typically, young and unencumbered by knowledge of how things are, they expect health care to work like other staples in their lives—Uber, Amazon, iPhones. Why wouldn't it? They want options. Unlike Researchers (discussed later), for whom choices represent the path to confidence in their decisions, Aspiring Shoppers just want to find best-fit products at prices that fit their budgets. They don't know how things work or why they don't. They have no sense that their expectations are crazy, because, well, they aren't.

The Quarterback

"I'm my own advocate," Andrea told me. "My husband's my advocate. We are the quarterbacks." In Chapters 7 and 9, I share her harrowing story of a bleak cancer diagnosis. When standard treatment protocols didn't work, the mother of three young children feared the worst. Andrea and her husband took charge of the process, seeking second and third opinions; investigating alternatives; and pursuing promising, if nonstandard, treatment approaches. Through their own navigation and extreme self-advocacy, Andrea got the information and treatment she needed and learned just how much effort being a health care consumer can require.

Are You a Quarterback?

Some people want to be told what to do when it comes to health care, and they do it. Not Quarterbacks. They recognize that no one will look out for their interests better than they will. They have the capacity to see the whole playing field and are not afraid to direct their own care. Like Organizers, they can stay on top of health care complexity and take self-reliance to a whole new level. Quarterbacks understand and accept that they are the drivers of their health care journeys.

The Avoider

Ruby hated going to the doctor. She hated even interfacing with the medical system. "I made sure I had health insurance and then strenuously avoided going to the doctor for 15 years," she told me. Profiled in Chapters 6, 7, and 9, Ruby was a heavy smoker and didn't want to be lectured about the damage she knew she was doing to her body. Culturally, she had been raised on medical care via one of the first HMOs (health maintenance organizations), which did not require much navigation. The HMO set the rules and created a sort of one-stop shop, for better or worse. Also, Ruby just wasn't ready to manage adult situations like choosing doctors and proactively managing one's health. Conveniently, she married an active health care consumer and gladly relies on him to manage their family's health care details. She'd rather not think too much about it or engage with it at all.

Are You an Avoider?

Please don't talk to Avoiders about doctors, health care, medical bills, or anything in a 10-mile radius of those things. If they can get away without ever going to the doctor, they will try. Expect them to show up in the emergency room on death's door before they'd go get a checkup. If a family friend or acquaintance can write them a necessary prescription, they'll go that route. If what they need requires a doctor visit, they'll probably wait it out as long as possible.

The Researcher

Louisa is a Researcher through and through. She shares her experience in Chapter 9. Suffering from a treatment-resistant infection, she was frustrated that her doctor was unable to come up with an effective treatment. Louisa took it upon herself to understand the scientific literature on her condition and would bring in academic studies to show her doctor that the treatment she had prescribed does not work. When I asked if Louisa researches all kinds of purchases, she focused on large, expensive items, but then added: "Not on the little stuff, but I am someone who looks at the ingredients on everything I buy." That's a Researcher.

Are You a Researcher?

Researchers are curious and skeptical. They don't blindly trust anyone, and they can find themselves in the uncomfortable position of educating their providers. They, more than other types, recognize that medicine involves art as well as science. That gives them confidence to question what they're told. They believe in their own ability to find and understand evidence. They want choices and to ultimately decide for themselves. Their decisions typically favor quality over cost savings, so long as there's some proof that the treatment will work.

The Sage

"Don't treat me like somebody who can't absorb information," Helen said. "I like explanations." At 92, Helen had built a trusting long-term relationship with her doctor, but she worried that he was beginning to see her as an "anxious old woman." When she chose a new doctor, it was to see someone who routinely dealt with "the typical declines of the elderly." She felt that she was betraying her previous doctor. Nonetheless, she wanted to be seen as an individual and to be taken seriously. She wanted information, options, and respect from her health care providers, whom she viewed as partners in her quest to live well and preserve her health as long as possible. Aware of her vulnerability and recognizing her mortality, Helen maintains her sense of humor about it. Read more about Helen and her peers in Chapter 15.

Are You a Sage?

Sages are older consumers, often considered "old old" rather than simply eligible for Medicare. They ask questions because they want to understand their situations—their bodies, their risks, and their options. They routinely make trade-offs, financial or otherwise. They recognize inevitable physical declines, but many remain cognitively sharp or at least capable of organizing and managing their financial and health care lives. They prefer to build true relationships with their health care providers and appreciate clinicians whom they know as people and vice versa. They prefer not to switch doctors or insurers, but if a compelling reason to arises—the doctor's own decline, a dramatic shift in health plan costs—they will evaluate the options and do what they must. Sages are attuned to details, organized, and responsible. They tend not to negotiate or unduly chase better financial deals. For many, health care costs are reasonable, benefiting from Medicare and generous retiree benefits, a mostly extinct phenomenon for the generations that follow. As old school as this segment can be—meticulously keeping records and managing their finances to the penny—they are also adapting to modern times. "Professor Google" is a key resource for many, even as they may not see the Internet as their friend. They represent a bridge between old values and modern methods. Raised at a time when frugality, modesty, and responsibility were prized values, they also appreciate modern technological and societal advances and have learned to benefit from them.

AT LEAST KNOW YOURSELF

The health care industry may be slow to recognize consumer purchasing power or to deploy sophisticated marketing and segmentation techniques that would help them better understand and reach different types of health care consumers. But consumers themselves can—and should—recognize their own styles, preferences, and needs. At least by knowing yourself, you can find services and providers that suit you. If you can vote with your feet and your wallet, the industry will have to follow.

PART TWO

The Consumer Manifesto

5

How Much Will This Cost?

How to find—and read—the health care price tag

Rosemary thought her husband's vasectomy was going to be covered; that's how she talked him into it. "We don't have to pay anything," she told him. Rosemary is unusually well informed about health insurance benefits, having worked for several years at a health insurance company before staying home with her two young children. Still, she was mistaken. "When the bill came for $500, he was none too pleased."

If a health insurance veteran gets surprised like this, how can anyone else expect to know what their health care is going to cost?

In Rosemary's case, she was confident she was correct. "I fought for a while. I asked for supervisors and whatnot, because I was reading the policy." That policy covered procedures related to family planning 100%. "This is a family planning-related procedure," she argued. "You get it to prevent pregnancy. That's the only reason you get a vasectomy."

Rosemary pressed the point until she learned the doctor who did the procedure billed it as a surgery because he performed it in an operating room. If he had done the vasectomy in an office, it would have been completely covered. Rosemary called a former colleague still working at the health plan she had left. "They're ripping you off," the colleague said. "It should not be billed as a surgery." But, learning that the procedure took place on the surgical floor, he revised his assessment. "Well, then you probably have to pay for it."

Rosemary can laugh about it, to a degree. "We have the luxury of it not being a make-or-break situation," she admitted. "I can't imagine what it must feel like if you literally cannot afford to pay this bill. I was just doing it . . . on principle. I didn't think we should be paying this bill."

Rosemary's experience illustrates a major obstacle to consumer shopping in health care: the lack of price transparency. It also offers a glimpse into why creating price transparency is so challenging: the same product can be billed in multiple ways, each with different price implications. Even if consumers think they understand the price, these nuances can change the picture entirely, without their knowledge—let alone genuine consent—ahead of time.

If you don't know what things will cost, how can you make informed choices and reasoned trade-offs?

WHAT PRICE?

The solution to price opacity seems simple—just publish the price. But what *is* the price of a health care service? I once asked my colleagues who negotiated provider contracts and payment terms, "Why don't we just publish prices?" I imagined the good press we would get for being first to take such an approach, not to mention consumer appreciation for clear and open communications. My colleagues, though, must have imagined endless angry phone calls from contracted hospitals and doctors demanding to know why we had exposed such sensitive information.

After recovering from their shock at my outrageous suggestion, my colleagues surfaced a more practical concern. "What price?"

Health care pricing is not only proprietary—our contracts may not even have allowed such disclosure—but also convoluted and intricately negotiated between hospitals, doctors, and health plans, with variation by provider, service, and insurance type. Like an airline ticket, the consumer's price depends on many factors, such as specific codes, key words, and which identifier the doctor uses on the bill. Has the consumer met his or her deductible? What copayment applies to that specific provider or treatment or setting where the treatment happens? As Rosemary learned, where a procedure takes place matters. For her, the location within a facility made the difference between a $500 out-of-pocket liability and 100% coverage.

Pricing complexity is just the tip of the iceberg. Underneath the nuanced rules and cautious corporate stances lies a deeper challenge: in many cases, no one really knows the price in the first place.

SETTING PRICES WITHOUT KNOWING THE COSTS

Price, in theory, relates to cost. Most businesses set their prices by adding a margin on top of their costs, or they base prices on the market's willingness to pay, assuming they can cover their costs.

The truth in health care is that almost no one knows the true costs of delivering services, making it difficult to set and communicate clear and rational pricing. Pat Rocap, a cost management consultant at health data and analytics firm Health Catalyst, knows the intricacies of this challenge. From her vantage point deep inside health care cost systems, she confirmed that charges—"the amount asked by a provider for a health care good or service"[1]—often have little connection to the true cost of delivering that health care service.

Most providers, Rocap explained, allocate costs to different departments or cost centers based on ratios, such as a "cost-to-charge" ratio—the relationship between a provider's expenses and their charges. A patient's charges are then converted to costs by applying a set ratio to derive the cost rather than by building up the cost based on the labor, supplies, and other goods needed to deliver the service.

"They're pushing down all this overhead cost that they want you to show a margin with, and they're judging you by it, yet they're not updating the standards of how you're getting costs, based on actual data and consumption." Costs, then, are calculated by allocation, regardless of what was actually spent in the cost center. "It's not the true cost," Rocap explained.

Costs are reverse engineered—derived based on set ratios rather than calculated on actual expenses. Those ratios, in turn, are set based on approximations and estimations. Using this standard method, health care costs are not calculated based on the real components of a service's or procedure's cost but rather on overall overhead costs allocated to individual cost centers. "It gives you no insight on how to find waste or how to find variation," Rocap said.

Again, costs have often been calculated in relation to charges rather than based on consumption or expenses incurred. Calling this process circular feels like an understatement.

Ratios used to calculate costs often come from one-time cost studies that themselves used historical charges, not necessarily actual resource usage. Once set, they are rarely, or infrequently, revisited. "I have seen some accounting systems not even updated for several years," Rocap said. As the initial studies get more out of date, the cost allocations can get more out of whack and less related to true, current costs. Over time, resource consumption naturally shifts, but if resource allocations do not, allocations mask true financial performance. Not only do inaccurate cost bases persist, but their distortions are also perpetuated and amplified over time. Services may appear more or less costly than they truly are. Prices set on distorted cost assumptions only get less accurate over time.

Though providers may claim to use activity-based costing accounting methods in which resource consumption along with indirect costs are assigned to activities to derive estimated costs of those activities,[2] Rocap debunks that claim. "Once again, it's just a relative value that you've assigned to something based on a one-time study that you might have done years ago."

If doctors and hospitals don't know their real costs, on what basis are they setting health care prices? Peeking into health care's accounting underbelly makes it hard to imagine health care prices could possibly be rational.

It also explains deeper roots of price opacity. Without knowing true costs, prices are set in a circular, arbitrary way. In turn, prices are convoluted and hard to publish in a consumer-friendly way. Were consumers to ask why the prices are what they are, it would be almost impossible to provide good answers.

Rocap's work aims to bring clarity to the accounting muck at the bottom of health care cost accounting. Her employer, Health Catalyst, offers analytic tools and improved cost reporting to thousands of clinics, hospitals, and provider systems. Working with health care providers to help them implement and understand cost reporting—using their real costs—still seems relatively novel in the industry.

Unleashing what should be basic data allows providers to examine waste in their practice and make operational changes. For example, Rocap described a group of surgeons that more critically examined how many surgical supplies they really needed to use. They realized the cost implications of opening a new stapler when stitching up patients after surgery; reloading the stapler took an extra step but saved significant dollars. Once they understood the data, they were able to identify and reduce waste in their practices.

Reducing waste in health care reduces costs, which, in turn, can help reduce prices for patients. But most doctors and hospitals do not yet have this kind of cost visibility. Rocap's assessment of the situation was bleak, unless you're measuring room for improvement. "I think you're going to find that 99 percent are probably using an old approach or none at all."

ANTICIPATORY CONFUSION

Consumer confusion over health care prices starts long before patients receive surprise bills and even before they get to the doctor's office. When people are choosing and using health insurance—discussed more extensively in Chapters 11, 12, and 13—it can be hard to figure out what care will cost based on one's benefits.

Gregg, a freelance musician in his early 60s not yet eligible for Medicare, was trying to choose a health plan during the Affordable Care Act open enrollment. Without clear price information, he was confounded. "I only had one drug that I was taking," he said. "There was no one that could answer what the cost would be, which to me seemed kind of outrageous because my situation is really rather simple. . . . It seemed like I had to make a decision without the information that I need."

He is not alone.

"I am just concerned that I'm going to go to the doctor and I'm going to have to pay a lot," Bella, a Millennial, explained why she had not been to the doctor since signing up for her own health insurance for the first time after losing access to her parents' plan. "I know I can look at my plan and see how much a doctor visit costs, but I just am worried that I'm going to get there and not actually be covered."

Lack of clarity and consumer confidence in health care pricing may explain why cost-sharing with consumers has not turned most people into smart shoppers. If you can't figure out the cost, how can you make rational choices to maximize economic value?

PRICE TAGS, DELAYED

Even if you think you know the cost based on your benefits, bills can still surprise you. Worse, it can take a long time to gather the full cost picture. Art's story illustrates the challenge of thinking you're buying one service and then having multiple bills straggle in, often long after the procedure itself occurs.

When Art learned that he needed sinus surgery for strep and staph infections that had overtaken one side of his face—as described further in Chapter 9—he had no idea what the surgery would cost. Yet he didn't ask because he thought he knew. "I thought I had an $800 deductible," he explained. "I just misunderstood. That wasn't the case. My belief was that my max out-of-pocket was going to be $800."

Months after the surgery, bills started rolling in from different providers who had been involved in the procedure. "I got bills from three different places. I got the lab. I got the surgery center. I got the doctor. I got the anesthesiologist. It's probably $4,000 or $5,000 that I pay. I had no visibility into this before the surgery. I just get bills after the fact."

Art's surprise was compounded by feeling he had already paid one bill.

I'm good. I'm not expecting any more bills at that point because I paid the doctor. He did the procedure. And then you start getting all these other bills from labs and everything else. You don't know about it. . . . The doctor knows these other services are going to be used. I, as a consumer, don't actually know what services he's going to use. . . . I could ask, but I consider myself a reasonably educated person. It didn't even cross my mind that his bill was not going to be inclusive of the five [subcontractors] that he was going to use in the process.

What had the surgeon discussed with him regarding costs? "Nothing."

The chaotic, haphazard nature of the billing was particularly frustrating. "I'm getting bills from ten different places. There appears to be no single point of accountability." He had no way to anticipate his total cost.

It seemed to Art to be no one's responsibility to organize or disclose the costs. "Nobody lays out and says, 'Just so you know, you're going to get four bills. You'll have one from the surgery center, one from this, one from this, one from this.' There's nobody who seems to be incentivized to communicate."

Not generally a fan of government mandates, Art thought one might be needed to clearly assign responsibility for cost disclosures. "There should be somebody there who lays it out. . . . Somebody has to say 'Before you sign up for this procedure, here's what your costs are going be,' or 'Here's what we expect them to be.'"

Other countries have developed better approaches to price transparency. Australia, where about half the population buys private insurance on top of the universal public coverage, requires doctors and hospitals to provide consumers with estimates of their total financial liability for treatments or procedures and encourages open discussion of costs.[3] In 2006, almost one in five Australians faced surprise bills for out-of-pocket liabilities, called "gaps," when they had a privately insured surgery.[4] In 2019, after implementing informed financial consent procedures more than a decade before, fewer than 15% of these surgeries had gaps at all. Australian consumers now face many fewer surprise bills when they do face gaps.[5]

In France, the government negotiates with doctors and hospitals on behalf of insurers, called "sickness funds," to set a single rate for any given service. Because the underlying pricing is so simple, it is easy, then, to post the rates.[6]

In Singapore, I snapped a photo of a price list on the check-in counter at a hospital I visited in 2013. The government now posts the average costs for all services online, searchable by procedure or topic.[7] One of the commonly cited limitations of price transparency is that you can't shop around when you're having a heart attack. But in Singapore, you can plan ahead and look up what your costs might be in case of emergency.

None of these approaches was at work for Art. Disillusioned by the layers of obstacles to price transparency, he admitted, "My whole idea around economics being transparent is so far from reality." To Art, health care is "the most dysfunctional, disjointed marketplace." The whole experience just seemed crazy. "I can't think of another situation where you would sign up for a major purchase without knowing [the price]."

NAVIGATING THE LABYRINTH

One reason it is so hard to disclose health care prices is that, often, the price depends on the outcome of the service. That would be like the price of a winter coat varying depending on how much it snowed after you bought it. You'd have to wait for the bill until after winter ended and the weather watchers calculated snow totals for the season.

Theo's story illustrates just such a scenario.

A 40-year-old writer and filmmaker based in Los Angeles, introduced in Chapters 3 and 4, Theo needed a colonoscopy to determine the cause of undiagnosed medical issues. Theo is a professional storyteller, and it was hard for me to not laugh while he regaled me with this tale. But it also made me want to scream.

Theo's doctor told him, "You need to get a colonoscopy at your young age because we need to rule out colon cancer." Theo called his insurance company to make sure the colonoscopy would be covered. They told him, "The procedure is 100% covered. Obviously, if they find polyps, and they have to remove polyps, that would be a different procedure. That will happen while you're under anesthesia, so you will have no say in that. They will just do it. And that's TBD, depending on what they need to do, whether or not that's covered and the amount that's covered."

Theo heard that as "I'm going under and when I wake up, I might have had three different procedures done, none of which [is] covered by my insurance company." He agreed to the procedure because, in his words, "If nothing is wrong, then the procedure is 100% covered. And if something is wrong, I'm really fucking glad they found it because I don't want to have colon cancer. So, that will be worth whatever I have to pay."

Theo continued his story and then stopped himself. "Oh, and there's something else. They said, basically, the doctor has to rent the space because the doctor doesn't have a place where he can do a colonoscopy. He leases from a clinic." The cheapest available space was $500.

"That was a fee my insurance company doesn't cover, the first thing they didn't cover," Theo clarified. "But then I was told that the anesthesia is often a claim that's rejected by the insurance company." (Why anesthesia would not be covered for a procedure requiring it—a procedure that the insurance company would approve—remains a mystery.) That charge would be $750. They would submit the claim, "but most likely my company was going to deny it because that's what they typically do," it was explained to Theo. "So that would be another $750 fee which I would have to pay."

The provider offered Theo an alternative to that uncertainty. "I could just pay them $250 up front for the anesthesia and there would be no claim." He decided to pay the $750 out of pocket—$500 for the clinic space rental and the $250 negotiated flat fee for anesthesia—once he understood the complexity of billing. It was a good deal for the clinic as well. "They're okay to only receive $250 anyway, that's probably what they would negotiate with the insurance company, and they saved the time negotiating by just telling me, 'What if you pay $250?' That saves them hours of time and it makes them the same money."

Unlike Art, Theo got visibility into all these fees and was offered a choice to accept the chaos or pay for certainty.

The story ended well for Theo. "It turns out that my colon is fine. There were no extra procedures needed. I woke up. I got off cheap at $750 for this procedure which was '100% covered.' Of course, that $750 does not count towards my deductible because none of it was through my insurance."

"If I had colon cancer, conversely, maybe it would have been worth it to get to my deductible faster. But whatever, if I had colon cancer, there's a lot more important things than $500 in my life. I'm healthy. And to find out that I'm healthy, I went through this whole labyrinth of things. So that's not what's wrong with me. I did all that to find out what isn't my problem."

FAILING GRADES

Given the underlying cost complexity, it may be no surprise that it's hard to find health care prices despite price transparency provisions in numerous state laws, components of the Affordable Care Act, and a federal rule[8] finalized in 2018 governing hospital price lists. The Pioneer Institute, which mystery-shopped 21 Massachusetts hospitals in 2017,[9] found that only 9 of the hospitals surveyed could provide price information within the state's required two days; 5 of the hospitals required consumers to offer a billing code for their desired procedure before giving that price. This result is especially disappointing in light of the fact Massachusetts had passed a health care price transparency law in 2012.[10]

Nationally, an annual report card on state health care price transparency[11] efforts gave only two states A grades in 2017; in all, 43 states received failing grades, the same number that had failed in the prior year.[12] What seemed heretical many years ago when I suggested exposing prices to consumers has become law, but it's not working yet.

What would "working" mean? And what impact might it have?

PRICE-COMPARING OUR WAY TO LOWER COSTS

Conventional health industry wisdom holds that if people know the cost of health services, they'll think twice about using them unnecessarily. They'll thoughtfully compare prices and, logically, choose the less expensive option.

In turn, doctors and hospitals, afraid of losing business—and of exposure and shame—would bring prices down, in line with what the newly transparent market will bear. Health care system-level costs—neatly aligned with consumers' financial incentives now that most people pay a meaningful portion of their health care costs via deductibles—will go down. This virtuous cycle is the whole idea behind consumer cost-sharing and why we all pay a bigger share of health expenses, even if we have "good insurance," than we would have a decade or so ago.

"I would want [health care] to become more of a free market where providers are thinking about the prices that are being put out there, and consumers are reacting accordingly," Sarah Michalczuk, told me. Michalczuk is CEO of predictaBill, a health care transparency start-up she founded after experiencing her own frustrating surprise medical bills and finding no good solutions for consumers trying to plan their health care costs in advance of incurring them. In researching this problem with consumers, Michalczuk found that some consumers perceive higher-priced care to be higher quality—though they expect "white-glove service" in return. Others felt paying more was not worth it and wanted ways to shop for better value. With greater transparency, Michalczuk anticipates shifting market prices as some providers angle for higher fees and others feel downward pricing pressure. "I could also see the free-market forces accelerating policy change," she said. Once the public can better understand health care pricing, perhaps they would demand more protections from unfair and irrational rates.

A friend of mine shared another lens into how price transparency could nudge prices down. "Lack of transparency feels like one of the reasons health costs must be so high," my friend posted to Facebook, after buying her own insurance when she became a self-employed consultant. She chose a plan with no prescription drug coverage. "I did the math and it cost more in premium to get the drugs covered than to pay out of pocket for them. So, I just shopped my prescriptions around, which I never did before because I had health insurance." Newly subject to health care price variation, she found that a prescription she had filled for about $60 at one major pharmacy chain, with an online coupon, cost $9 at another chain. On her previous employer-sponsored health plan, she had paid an $11.81 copayment for the same prescription. "If consumers don't pay out of pocket, they don't shop around, *and* providers make it really difficult to shop around—try getting your [doctor] to quote you actual prices *before* you have the [appointment]—why would our health care be optimized and a perfect market?"

THE LIMITS OF PRICE TRANSPARENCY

Despite the promise of price transparency efforts, results have been mixed. One study showed that people who used available price transparency tools had lower overall claims for lab tests, physician visits, and imaging, whether or not they personally benefited from the lower costs.[13] Yet other studies have shown that lower overall costs result not from people comparing prices and choosing lower ones but from their simply seeking less care overall.[14] (I explore the impact of cost-sharing and erosion of health insurance value further in Chapter 13.)

Researchers found no significant differences in what people on high-deductible plans paid for services compared with people on traditional plans in eight out of nine service categories.[15] Still another study found that use of a price transparency tool was actually associated with higher spending overall and out of pocket.[16]

Where price data are available, people support the concept but do not actually use the data. A large national survey found that though 72% of respondents thought comparing cost and/or quality of medical services would be good for the United States, only 13% had sought information about their out-of-pocket costs, and even fewer—just 3%—had compared costs across providers.[17] Other research shows 10% uptake of price transparency tools.[18]

Where people use price transparency tools, they still may not have a big impact on overall costs. Tal Gross, PhD, associate professor at Boston University's Questrom School of Business, pointed me to a study that showed the impact of a price transparency website was relatively minimal, yielding a 5% reduction in prices.[19]

One study found that 35%[20] of spending was on "shoppable" services, defined as services that are common and that consumers can research in advance to compare multiple providers, with available cost and quality data on which to base a selection.[21] The Health Care Cost Institute analyzed the same question using a more nationally representative sample and found 43% of services were shoppable, equivalent to $524 billion in health care spending.[22]

Reducing shoppable expenses by 5%, as Gross referenced, may not yield desired savings. On $3.5 trillion in national health expenditures annually, "That's still a lot of money," Gross said. "But it's not that big a deal." Price transparency is hard to argue against, so politically speaking, efforts to increase transparency seem "like a trivial thing to do, that's going to actually change nothing or not threaten anyone's income, at least not that much." To date, there is not a lot of evidence that price transparency dramatically changes behavior or solves the health care cost conundrum.

The solutions themselves may be, in part, to blame for the lackluster impact. NPR and *Kaiser Health News* profiled one drug price tool embedded in electronic health record systems and noted its limitations; not all pharmacy data were included, so this tool intended to help doctors prescribe lower-cost options worked for only half the patients.[23]

Implementation of a 2019 price transparency law[24] requiring hospitals to publish charges has been less than ideal; the lists can be hard to find and harder still to read and interpret.[25] Numerous ventures are providing price transparency—through crowdsourcing or partnerships with payers and/or providers. Few, however, cover all geographies or the full scope of health care services. These valiant efforts move price transparency in the right direction, but none has proven to be a holy grail.

Kevin McDevitt, director, social determinants of health at Spring Street Exchange, and former IT implementation manager at the Massachusetts Health Connector, reflected on poor transparency implementation. "There's a tendency when you say transparency to try to show everything. And the downside of that is then people get confused or overwhelmed and they don't digest the information." He argued, instead, for presenting the most important items in a clear way.

Professor Gross raised another potential obstacle to price transparency: collusion. "When prices are shrouded, then the price setters—the producers—don't quite know what everyone is charging," Gross explained, and lack of visibility into prices can keep prices lower as providers want to ensure they are competitive. "But then when prices are all public on a website, you could end up with a kind of tacit collusion." Lower-priced providers see competitor rates and want to earn as much. Once lower-cost providers adjust upward, they can monitor one another, and no one's likely to budge or not too dramatically. "It could make real collusion more feasible or it could make tacit collusion possible." Gross thinks price transparency, therefore, could result in unintended consequences. Yet, in retail markets, prices are on full display, and still competition thrives. Hospitals are competitive entities, vying for volume and likely to compete aggressively, including on price.

Cultural factors may also limit consumer willingness to choose lower-cost options even when the data are available. Dr. Heather Ross of Arizona State University suggested consumer attitudes about value are, themselves, potential obstacles to shopping based on price. "I don't think it's socially valued to say, 'I chose my doctor because they have the cheapest price.'" People are likely to interpret the lower price as "It must be the worst. Why would you want to choose the worst of anything for your health care?" Ross suggested consumer attitudes may follow the old maxim: "You get what you pay for."

SHARED IGNORANCE

Consumers' testimony illustrates the practical challenges of figuring out health care prices and of using that information to make smart, high-value choices.

"When I go to the doctor, and I go to have tests done, they never say, 'You're going to be responsible for this,'" Rosemary described her experience. "You find out six weeks later, which was fine when you basically never paid for it yourself, because you paid for your insurance, and that was it. But that just doesn't happen anymore."

Rosemary had recently been treated for what she was pretty sure was a gallstone. At the doctor's office, she described her pain, and they sent her to get blood tests and an ultrasound. "Never once did I see anything that said it might cost you this much. I signed something when I walked in agreeing to pay whatever my insurance won't pay, but never did I see anything that said [what that would be]. . . . And I guess I didn't ask either, because I don't even think they could answer the question."

Rosemary is probably right. Many doctors could not answer these questions and many don't want to; some were actually trained not to discuss or factor costs. Doctors typically don't set the price, as fee schedules are negotiated with health plans, usually at a health system level. Worse than not controlling the price, doctors often don't even know what the prices are.

In Chapter 3, I shared one private-practice psychologist's admission that he cannot tell patients what to expect—except in general terms—because he, himself, doesn't know what insurance will reimburse patients who pay his fees out of pocket.

Heather Ross revealed price information is no more clear to nurses. "Nurses have no idea how much—every time you pull another pack of gauze out of the cabinet for your patient, you have no idea what the patient is getting charged for that pack of gauze. It never enters in," she told me.

The culture of medicine has historically steered clinicians away from even acknowledging cost. "Cost is like the dirty little secret of health care, on both ends," Ross explained. She was trained to be agnostic to cost when prescribing medications and ordering tests. "In nursing education, there was almost no discussion of cost. Nursing is supposed to be this very ethically pure exercise. Cost feels like it's ethically problematic and not pure."

A colleague once told Ross, "I don't want to know how much anything costs. I only make decisions based on what's best for the patient. And if I know what the costs are, then it's ethically wrong for me to factor cost in, so I don't even want to know how much it costs." If cost considerations could cloud clinical judgment inappropriately, clinicians would violate their moral obligation, which is, according to Ross, "to prioritize quality and saving the life, curing the disease, optimizing the quality of my patient's life above all else."

Clinician reluctance to discuss costs—philosophically and because of lack of preparation for such discussions—may be generational and going out of style.[26] For example, virtually all medical schools require students to take courses that cover health care cost topics, and the American College of Physicians now offers free training modules on health care costs.[27]

A medical student we interviewed took the initiative to educate himself about costs by going to the drugstore with his patients in mind. "It wasn't until I started getting medical experience that I actually walked down the aisles and looked at [what things cost], even though I didn't have to. It was nice to know the prices of what the patients who I was working with in the future might have to incur. Because it always impressed me [when] my preceptors could tell the patient, 'I'm not going to prescribe this because it would probably be cheaper if you just go to CVS and get Tylenol for $2.89.' The patients were really at ease when he did that."

In a survey my Harvard Kennedy School research team and I conducted in 2019,[28] of 525 U.S. medical students who participated, 77% reported getting some formal training on health care cost topics. However, of those who had received formal training, only 45% reported getting trained on consumer-level cost topics, such as how to determine a patient's out-of-pocket costs or how to discuss costs with patients. Worse, only about one-third (36%) who had received formal cost-related training rated that training effective, and almost two-thirds of all survey respondents (64%) felt unprepared to discuss costs with patients. Medical schools may be realizing they need to train students on health care costs, but they have a lot of room to improve the effectiveness of that training.

Whether deliberate or genuine ignorance, doctors tend not to share cost information proactively or to open cost conversations with patients. Doctors often perceive that discussing costs will add significant time to already-rushed medical visits,[29] and as Ross suggested, it runs counter to traditional medical training and culture.

AFRAID TO ASK

The other side of providers' inability or unwillingness to discuss costs with patients is the patients' reluctance to ask about costs. Consumers report being uncomfortable raising cost concerns and may assume it is not okay to do so, though most report thinking or worrying about health costs regardless of their insurance status.[30] Rosemary admitted she didn't bother asking because she assumed the doctors wouldn't know. Heather Ross also noted it's rare for her patients to ask about costs. "Most patients certainly don't have a medical background to ask even about, 'Can I take this? And what's the pricing on it?' They just think, 'My doctor said I should do this, so this is what I should do.'"

Numerous consumers echoed this sentiment. "I just do what my doctors tell me to do," said Sophie, a working mother and self-described hypochondriac. "If they say I should see a specialist, I see a specialist. I don't really comparison-shop or anything like that. I just figure the finances will take care of themselves."

Paulette, a woman in her 60s, described the deep roots of consumer disempowerment. "We were brought up to never question doctors; they knew everything. . . . They have so much education, and who am I? I'm just a little nothing."

THE PATH TO PRICE TAGS

On the other hand, there are examples in some corners of health care where price disclosures are the norm—usually because patients pay all or a substantial portion of costs out of pocket—like mental health care and dentistry, discussed in Chapters 3 and 14, respectively. Another classic case is LASIK eye surgery, which replaced a procedure that in 1997 cost $8,000[31] and today can cost less than $2,000.[32] Because insurance didn't cover the procedure, providers competed on price to attract paying consumers. Technological advances enabled efficiency, but market force required it.

In Theo's colonoscopy story, his providers developed a transparent work-around rather than investing energy and time in submitting claims only to face near-certain insurance denials. Their solution likely resulted in comparable earnings for them and much less hassle for everyone involved.

In an adjacent sector, Rosemary described how her vet gets around the problem of uncertainty. When she brings her dog to get her teeth cleaned once a year, the vet discloses they may need to pull a tooth. Rosemary signs a form authorizing up to $150 in services, and they call her if it will cost more. The same thing happens when she leaves her car at the mechanic's shop. "But you never get that as a person."

Some people do get this level of transparency in some aspects of care, and more could. Concierge doctors and direct primary care providers—who typically charge membership fees directly to patients to avoid insurance rules—offer clear pricing. Others simply don't accept insurance, instead billing consumers directly. When their first child was born, Adam and his wife chose a pediatrician—described in Chapter 9—who does not accept any insurance. The first time they met with the pediatrician in her office, she gave the couple a worksheet and offered them options of paying for multiple visits up front at a 15% or 20% discount, or they could pay for each visit. "It was all printed out on a sheet," Adam described. "You could do the math on it. It was certainly helpful to see that in one place."

The pediatrician provided bills with insurance codes that they could submit for reimbursement. "But it's on us to file." The pediatrician spends at least an hour with the family at each visit and explained, "If I took insurance, that would get cut in half easily because I would spend half of that time dealing with all the crap that comes with having to deal with insurance companies. . . . I would much rather sit with you here for an hour and have a leisurely conversation about your kid, rather than have to hustle you out after 25 minutes to get the next person in so that I can deal with all the red tape." They got some reimbursement from their insurer but they were willing to pay regardless. They have had no surprises and no regrets about their decision.

Common in these examples of transparency is the absence of health insurers muddying the price signals. Direct transactions between consumers and their providers make clear that transparent pricing schemes are possible—just like in psychotherapy—where there's a will and no intermediary.

Choosing providers who recognize the importance of price transparency and simplicity—and deliver a better approach—is one powerful way consumers can help improve price transparency. The more popular these practices become, the more the industry will take notice. Absent switching to such a provider, the single most important thing consumers can do to both gain insight into their health costs and inspire broader systemic change is to ask two questions: First, what will this cost me? And, second, why?

1. What will this cost me?

The best way for consumers to help create a culture of price transparency is to demonstrate willingness to discuss costs. Say, "Can you tell me how much I should expect to pay?" or "What will my portion of the bill likely be?" Always ask, even if you think you know, like Rosemary and Art mistakenly did. Ask even if you feel shy or uncomfortable. Ask even if you think your doctor doesn't know the answer. Increasingly, consumers bear out-of-pocket costs because of deductibles. It is, therefore, increasingly common for consumers to ask what things cost. It is eminently reasonable to want to know. And it is increasingly untenable for providers not to have specific, concrete answers. A steady stream of consumer inquiries will become a flood the industry can no longer ignore.

2. Are there any other costs I might have to pay?

In the quest to ask what health care services will cost, it may be necessary to ask in a few different ways. Eliza, a 29-year-old woman, said she always asks about cost up front "as a result of experiences where I've gotten a bill and been totally surprised by how much it is." She had recently discussed the cost of a procedure she needed with the doctor's billing office. When she got the bill for more than they had discussed, she was shocked. "We had been talking about one aspect of what was happening as opposed to the whole procedure."

Like Art getting bills from the various subcontractors to his surgeon, Eliza's bill included components about which she hadn't thought to ask. "It's just made me more paranoid," she said. "I started to be way more vigilant about understanding what [things cost] up front."

It's hard to ask about costs you can't even imagine, but given consumer experiences with surprises, it's good practice to ask one more question about cost than you think is necessary, such as, "Is there anything else that I could be charged for?" Worst case, having asked for a thorough accounting of all potential costs, you'll have a basis for arguing later if you get a surprise bill after the fact.

Jason, a start-up executive insured on a very high-deductible plan that he buys for himself, is not shy in asking about health care costs. But he can't always even tell what services he is getting, making it nearly impossible to jump in to ask about costs. He has even had this experience at the dentist, despite Jason's sense that dental costs are based on more set fees. "I guarantee you I've never paid the same thing for a dentist appointment twice. They will whip out the X-ray machine and then two minutes later, you just spent $80 that you didn't know you were going to pay. I've just gotten really good at being like, 'Whoa! Hold up with that X-ray machine. I don't need that.' But at a doctor's appointment, it's less easy to tell."

3. Why?

"Why?" may be a harder question to ask, as people may not want to seem difficult or oppositional. Why will also likely be a much harder question to answer. But it is the *why* behind health care pricing that really needs addressing. Your doctor probably did not set the price and could not justify it even if he or she knows what it is. But shouldn't your doctor be able to address this fundamental and legitimate question that may directly impact your ability to follow his or her clinical recommendations? Shouldn't doctors stand behind the value of their services?

Even though Jason routinely asks about costs, he can't always make sense of the responses. "You know what's weird is that the prices are always different," Jason noted. "It's almost like it depends on the mood of the person at the front desk at the time. I have literally had the same person at the same front desk quote me wildly ridiculous rates for the exact same service at different times. And I don't know if it's because their policy changed and their price changed, or if it's just random."

That's not good enough, not when you're paying the bill. So ask away. Ask the doctor. Ask the receptionist. Ask your health insurer. Ask until you start hearing answers that make sense.

Price transparency solutions need to aim deeper than opening a window onto the current convoluted pricing system. Visibility into a mess isn't likely to bring about transformational consumerism, and efforts to do so haven't worked. Rather, pricing ought to be set with an audience in mind— the consumer. Consumers don't care, and should not need to know, which billing code commands higher reimbursement or which tax identification number the provider should use when billing for a procedure to minimize the consumer's financial obligation. Consumers should demand more than a preview of their likely costs; they also want and should get options for how to get the best price or at least to understand what value they may get for paying more.

6

Can You Do Any Better on the Price?

Negotiating our way to lower health care costs

"I'll give you $6," my fearless friend Troy offered the merchant in a stall in Morocco's Fez bazaar, which stretches and turns for what feels like miles, lined with everything from rugs and T-shirts to spices and delicacies like sheep's heads and pigeon pies.

"$10, come on," bartered the merchant. The item in question was a ceramic bowl small enough to carry home, where it would leave behind the vast sea of like-items to stand on its own, a unique treasure stateside. The price tag read $12.

"Nah. You know what?" Troy countered. "I'll give you $4."

Wait, what?

"No, man. I've got kids." The merchant pleaded. "Ok, ok, I'll give it to you for $8. That's my best price."

"I'm not sure I even want it. Maybe I'd give you $2." Troy shifted his weight, on the go, as if this discussion was about to end badly for the merchant, whose eyes widened with fear. This American was serious. And a little nuts.

"Ok, ok! $4!" the merchant cried. Please don't leave me without a sale, his tone shrieked.

Outside in the maze once again, Troy patted the ceramic piece wrapped in newsprint, safely tucked into the messenger bag slung across his torso, and smirked. "And that, my friends, is how it's done."

Years later, as a health plan executive negotiating contracts with pomp-
ous vendors already certain of our business and unaccustomed to making
concessions, I tried the corporate equivalent of Troy's bazaar haggling,
countering with something less than the terms on the table. My colleagues
would hold their breath—or perhaps roll their eyes—when my response to
a vendor's counterproposal was worse than my original offer. "It can't hurt
to ask," I'd coach less-confident negotiators. It didn't always work, but
when it did, I saw firsthand that fear of loss is a powerful motivator.

I'm certain Troy did not care about the $2 difference in price, but I can't
say definitively what made him so bold in the bazaar: an underlying self-
confidence, a desire to entertain us with his antics, a quest to win? He is a
serial entrepreneur, born salesman, and textbook extrovert; negotiating is
like a native language for him.

I tried to emulate Troy in a business setting where I had otherwise
reached an impasse. I tried not to fear being mocked, offending the vendor,
or losing the deal. Had the ceramics merchant stood firm, Troy could have
walked into any other stall and bought a similar item from someone else,
now more certain of the item's true value. Or he could have come back and
paid the vendor his price if he could not find a better alternative; that merchant would still take his money. In the corporate case, I most likely could
have reverted to the vendor's prior demands. Though people in movies and
TV shows sometimes storm out of a negotiation if the other party asks for
a concession, that does not happen too often in real life; I've certainly never
seen it. Trying and failing to get a better deal need not be the end of the
world, nor even the end of that deal.

FIXED-PRICE SOCIETY

Most Americans loathe negotiating. The car company Saturn used to
advertise set prices—no need to bargain—as a selling point. Now, increasingly popular car-buying apps and websites obviate haggling altogether.
My own introverted husband hid while sending me down a dusty row of
Hong Kong's jade market to negotiate for some small treasure he wanted.
He knew the custom was to bargain and didn't want to foolishly pay the
inflated list price. He just didn't want any part of the process of bartering
and couldn't even bear to watch.

Americans don't negotiate, and we have our reasons. For one, American
retailers are sophisticated, efficient, and increasingly data driven. Imagine
waiting in a grocery store line while each customer haggled over the total
cost of their items. That inefficiency creates a transaction cost for both
buyer and seller; it just makes no sense to take the time to negotiate for
small-dollar items. Retailers are moving in the opposite direction, embrac-
ing self-checkout registers and, even better, sensors and scanners that

identify what you bought and automatically charge your account when you leave the store; you'll never have to stop to check out at all. Moreover, in large retailers, prices and promotions are typically set strategically at a corporate level, and store staff usually have little authority to lower prices. Those same clerks are usually paid hourly whether they make a sale or not, so they don't have an incentive to deal.

Culturally, American aversion to negotiating runs deep and in many directions. Most Americans would never even test for flexibility in store prices. Shoppers have been trained that prices clearly marked are firmly set. And American retail is like an extension of our democracy. Price tags apply to everyone equally—we may all have different means, but if you can pay the price, the item can be yours. Set prices are easier and seem fair.

America's fixed prices are said to have originated in 1823 at Alexander Stewart's New York dry goods store. Packaged goods with brand names were rising, bolstered by advertising and consumer perception that these goods were higher quality and more hygienic. To relatively new generations of Americans trying to differentiate themselves from even newer immigrants, negotiating was a symbol of poverty and lower social class. Buying fixed-priced goods allowed these groups to signal that they belonged in American society, that they had willingly paid their fair share, and that they were not trying to get something for nothing[1]—a cardinal sin against American industriousness and entrepreneurial spirit.

Ironically, what may have stemmed from a form of social climbing in which people sought to distinguish themselves as belonging more than perceived outsiders, embrace of fixed prices is also seen as a manifestation of American values of egalitarianism, fairness, and a uniquely American friendliness or social congeniality. In keeping with our self-image as members of a polite, civilized society, Americans don't want to offend anyone, appear cheap, or seem greedy. Gretchen Herrmann's research on American garage sale negotiations found that 29% of buyers surveyed cited not wanting to be rude or obnoxious as the reason they did not try to negotiate.[2]

In Kyoto's Nishiki market, a seemingly infinite, covered arcade of food stalls selling Japanese bites like baby octopus stuffed with a hard-boiled egg yolk and rice ball skewers coated in oozing sweetened soy glaze, I asked my host about Japanese bargaining culture or lack thereof. Though this market had the chaotic, crowded feeling of markets in parts of the world where haggling is the norm, our guide paid for items like she would in a store. "In Osaka, they are businesspeople; maybe they bargain," she told me. "In Kyoto, people come from a high class, and maybe we are proud." Here, too, negotiating seems reflective of socioeconomic class. In this city filled with descendants of aristocracy, it was just not done.

Tough negotiations—in which sellers may concede initially and then stand firm without any joviality—connote, to many Americans, aggression, unfairness, and greed. In some cultures, tough negotiators successfully extract higher prices from buyers, but Americans don't tend to like that style. Herrmann's research includes stories of sellers who shut down their sales and donate goods rather than deal with aggressive negotiators, and others who reported being offended or insulted by tough bargainers seeking to squeeze the last dimes out of a price.

Sellers who haggle as a rule in the United States typically occupy professional roles—mainly in sales of large-ticket items—that are perceived as shady and untrustworthy or at least primarily concerned with their own financial gain. This view of negotiating is grounded in a common belief that bargaining is a zero-sum game; the more *you* get, the less there is for *me*. Yet I remember a business school lesson that defined the most successful negotiators as those who can make the pie bigger rather than viewing the pie as fixed and grabbing the biggest possible slice for themselves.

As uncomfortable as most Americans are with negotiation, consumption itself defines American culture. We shop for fun, like a national pastime. Many Americans eagerly chase sales for sport, hunting online for the best price. But haggling over price is simply not part of the game. Whereas paying less for an item we want can feel like an accomplishment—a testament to our own cleverness—somehow *asking* to pay less feels more like seeking a handout. Ruggedly individualistic, self-reliant Americans just do not do that.

Not to mention, how would consumers know what these goods are worth? We often have little visibility into what things should cost, so we are anchored by the price tag. Americans tend to assume a relationship—a rational one—between the price and value of an item. A discount off the fixed price seems like a win, without recognition that there may have been no rational basis for the price to begin with. Still other consumers would rather pay more to signal status. "Look what I can afford to buy," high-end designer goods advertise on our behalf. Bargaining has no place in that "more-is-better" mentality.

Finally, some research suggests the counterintuitive notion that the more bargainers participate in a market, the more prices will increase. Though more competition is thought to put pressure on sellers to keep costs low, in fact, sellers may actually raise list prices to allow for more bargaining while protecting their financial gains. Those new to bargaining benefit from lowering their costs compared to prices they had previously not negotiated, but those already in the market who always negotiate and those in the market who continue to not negotiate pay more, anchored by higher list prices.[3]

WE HAVE OUR REASONS

Given the general discomfort with negotiation, it's no wonder that Americans tend not to negotiate in health care, a sector approaching 20%

of the U.S. economy. In my consumer research, we asked if people had ever negotiated health care prices. Not only did they generally say "no," some admitted they "didn't even know that was an option." I was surprised that for some my question felt like a suggestion.

"I should, I guess," Tessa, a 40-year-old, stay-at-home mom of three, told me sheepishly. I spoke to her by phone while she made her way to pick up her youngest child from kindergarten. Though I assured her my question didn't imply judgment, the gregarious former social worker with self-deprecating humor beat herself up a little. "I just think there probably is room for that and I never have. I'm terrible at that."

Jason, the 35-year-old tech start-up executive introduced in Chapter 5, said, "Maybe I will. I just never thought about it." When I met him at an outdoor restaurant on a windy fall day, he looked quintessentially preppy, with close-cropped hair and a nubby fleece over his button-down shirt and jeans. As much as he looked the part of privilege, Jason bought his own health insurance and still pays out of pocket for most of his health care because of a high deductible, which he has never met. Resourceful in nosing out the cheapest way to get the care he needs, Jason never considered negotiating outright. "It's soul-sucking, because the system's not set up for that." Not to mention, most Americans are not set up for that either.

Not everyone's avoidance of negotiating results from failure of imagination. In some cases, it may reflect a sense of powerlessness. Emily, a public relations professional in her 30s with sleek brown hair and a shy laugh, faced a delicate situation. At the time of our interview, she was deciding whether to switch to her husband's health insurance, basing her decision on the cost of her upcoming in vitro fertilization procedures under either plan. She had found her way to a sought-after fertility specialist in New York City and the provider's fee would not be negotiable. "The way the clinic laid it out for me was, 'We're doing the best we can and we're submitting things and we have special deals with certain pharmacies and we're getting you the best price that we can.' I don't mean to liken it to a car salesman, but it is kind of like, 'You're robbing me blind here, I can't charge any less. It's just not feasible for our practice.'"

Unlike Troy in the Moroccan bazaar, this was not a game. Emily did not want to shop around. Though she systematically compared each facet of cost, tearing up, she betrayed the raw emotion of infertility. The stakes were high and the goods highly specialized. "I know there's a line of people waiting to work with him," she said. "I don't feel like I necessarily have the leeway or leverage to say, 'You know, $15,000 wouldn't be so bad, right?' He's not knocking on my door. I'm knocking on his."

Sharing this sense of futility was Sean, a graduate student who was aware that negotiating could lower health costs. "I have read some articles that that is more possible than people may know, but I had no idea that could work."

Despite his education and prior job working with expert economists, Sean felt ill prepared to try. "I don't know enough about the system to know when you have good leverage to do that and when you don't."

For others, like Sophie, anxiety is the obstacle to negotiating health care prices. When Sophie and her husband moved from Manhattan to Dallas for her husband's job, they needed to buy a car and followed guidance they had read in *Consumer Reports*. "They urge you to really push back and negotiate hard." The first-time car buyers dutifully sought quotes from local dealerships and national websites. "We brought all of those quotes to the dealership where we wanted to buy our car and they knocked a couple of thousand dollars off the price. It was an amazing deal. I don't know why we don't do that with health care. I think it's because there's not that same sense of anxiety and panic around having a car as there is around 'what will this test result show?'" In Sophie's health care encounters, the mental energy required to negotiate effectively is otherwise devoted to worrying about her health.

Clara did not negotiate for fear the quality of her care would suffer. A 98-year-old in the midst of costly dental work when I interviewed her in her living room, Clara spoke with a lisp as she awaited the final stage of her dental implant process. I asked if she had negotiated beyond the modest "senior discount" her dentist had proactively offered. "I didn't bargain," she said in her thick Brooklyn accent. "I didn't want him to cut corners. I figured if this is what it is, how could you bargain with the dentist?" She feared he would send her to "the clinic"—presumably a less-desirable provider—if she dared ask for a better deal. Like the garage-sale buyers in Herrmann's study, Clara didn't want to offend her dentist—as aggressive garage-sale buyers in Hermann's study had offended sellers—and risk paying some imagined consequence.

Still others did not negotiate because prices quoted seemed fair. "I know the stories of people negotiating down their huge hospital bills with insurers and hospitals, but I haven't been faced with bills like that, so I haven't felt the need," Eric shared. He's lucky. Patient financial responsibility after insurance leaves off increased by more than 50% between 2012 and 2017, leading to $2.6 billion of uncompensated care (i.e., bills that patients cannot or do not pay).[4] Chapter 5 explores the messy roots of health care pricing, which may help explain why pricing can be so opaque. For Eric, though, "either it's been completely covered or it's been what I thought to be a reasonable charge." How did he determine the charges' reasonableness? He laughed. "That's a good question, I don't know. . . . How *do* I know I'm getting a fair rate?" Stumbling, he finally offered that the absolute dollars were not crushing, and his insurance paid a portion. Fair enough.

Eric isn't alone in finding small dollars not worth negotiating. Hazel, the small-business owner with an optimistic outlook introduced in Chapter 4, does not want to spend time fighting with insurance or arguing medical bills. "How much is it worth it to sit down and spend the whole day matching up all these bills to all the communications for my insurance company? Do I really want to spend my whole day doing that? Probably not." She pondered the value of her time, easily quantifiable to a graphic designer managing her own firm. "Is it worth it if I find they made a mistake and I end up saving us $100? I guess deep down I feel like it wasn't worth it. . . . Truthfully, there are only so many hours in the day, and the days go by so quickly." A skiing fanatic living in a mountain resort town, she has better ways to spend her time.

Gregg, the musician introduced in Chapters 2 and 5, made similar calculations though his income is modest and inconsistent. He read online that his dental insurance covered fillings. Deep in the fine print of the plan details, though, he realized they only covered mercury fillings. "I haven't had mercury fillings in like 30 years." He called to complain that they had misrepresented the coverage. "I said, 'I think this is so fraudulent because nobody gets those kind of fillings anymore.' And they had nothing to say." Nonetheless, he didn't fight that hard. "They were covering $80 instead of $180 or something like that," Gregg explained. "And to get into some huge thing over $100 just seemed like I couldn't waste my time." Negotiating takes time and effort, not just imagination and confidence. The juice must be worth the squeeze.

Avoiding aggravation also outweighs the economic value for Theo, an irreverent writer and filmmaker in Los Angeles, described in previous chapters. Theo declared, "I'm not a negotiator. If somebody says I owe them $450, just the kind of person I am, I'm like, 'I owe them $450.' It's a bummer. It's a bummer that it worked out this way. It's a bummer that my doctor sent my labs to someone who's out of network, but I'm not going to call my insurance company to have a two-hour conversation that ultimately makes me super angry and still in debt $450."

The most unique reason I heard for not negotiating came from Ingrid, a public-school teacher in California who teaches children in lower-income school districts. She almost seemed to take offense at the question. "I wouldn't negotiate because I'm not low income. I don't need a sliding scale. That's just what they're charging." Like the early Americans proud to pay the new-fangled fixed prices as a sign of status, Ingrid associated bargaining with poverty and lower social class.

NEGOTIATION HAPPENS

People do negotiate health care costs, more often than even they realize. Websites like Healthcare Bluebook exist to help consumers negotiate health care prices, and *Consumer Reports*, long a trusted source on all sorts of consumer purchases, offers consumers guidance on successfully negotiating health care bills.[5] And it seems that each year, media outlets publish tips on getting better prices in health care or personal accounts of having successfully done so.[6]

Ingrid herself described visits to her childhood dermatologist who diagnosed melanoma when she was 30. Fair and freckled, she is a child of the 1970s when parents were less militant about sunscreen. When Ingrid moved across the country and switched insurance, she still returned home for annual skin checks. The first year on new insurance, she told the doctor, "I'm paying out of pocket. Can you just not make it too much?" The doctor agreed. "Sure, I'll check this box." But then, "one year, he forgot, and it was like $400 or $500 and that was too much. So, I emailed him and said, 'I think you forgot to check the box,' and he fixed it." Now, every year she reminds the dermatologist up front that she is paying out of pocket. What box did Ingrid's doctor check to lower her out-of-pocket expense? Perhaps this doctor's office had a self-pay designation that automatically triggered a lower fee or an informal system in which the doctor signaled the billing department to charge Ingrid less. Whether the box was literal or figurative, it was real to Ingrid—the key to getting a lower price, like a button that unlocks a secret door or a password that allows entry to an exclusive club. Once she knew the code, she wasn't shy about using it to her financial benefit. That sure sounds like negotiating to me.

More often, however, I found people had negotiated after they got a bill that felt unfair. George, a wry New York City finance executive, had such a story. At a family event, George's brother-in-law had suggested George—in his 40s—get a full cardiac exam from a cardiologist he recommended. George looked up the doctor, liked his credentials, and called to make an appointment. He explained he was a new patient and told the receptionist he had Aetna. "Great, please show up 20 minutes early for your 11:00 A.M. appointment," the receptionist said. George did not ask about the cost but figured he would hit his deductible because of other tests he had gotten that year. This exam should effectively be subsidized.

Once at the visit—having arrived 20 minutes early, in keeping with his respectful, responsible style—he filled out the paperwork and let the receptionist take a copy of his Aetna card. Then he waited for the doctor. And waited—for an hour and a half. After the exam, so annoyed by the delay and late getting back to work, George left without discussing the bill. Accustomed to getting bills for services subject to his high deductible, he didn't give it much thought.

Two weeks later, a $2,700 bill arrived. That's when George looked on Aetna's website and learned this doctor was not in their network, which meant George would pay 100% instead of sharing the cost with insurance after he satisfied his deductible. George is even-tempered with a dry wit that can make it hard to tell when he's made a joke, but the receptionist's lack of proactive transparency made him furious. Still, he relayed his fury calmly to me. "She could have simply told me that he's not in the network and I would have made a call as to whether it's worthwhile to spend the money." George didn't keep his frustration to himself. "I called them and I said, 'Listen, I didn't know that you weren't in network. Of course, I could have checked that, but I would have at least appreciated a heads up that you weren't.'"

After venting over bad service, he went on, ever rational: "I view my hourly time to be as valuable as the doctor's." George's hourly rate as a Manhattan finance executive is probably at least as valuable as the doctor's. "So you could have called ahead of time to let me know that he was late." The receptionist apologized, and George went in for the ask. "Given all of that," he politely proposed, "I would like the doctor, if you don't mind, to give some consideration to a discount off of the $2,700 price." She put George on hold, returned, and offered, "How about $1,800?"

George took the deal. "At that moment, honestly, I just wanted to move on." He recognized he could have gotten a few hundred dollars more off had he made a counteroffer, but it was just not worth it to him. He had always expected to pay something. The negotiated rate fell within those expectations.

George treated the experience like a business encounter. The doctor's time is worth something, as is his own. The doctor's office had not prepared him for the costs, nor delivered the experience George had expected. In that context, negotiating a fairer rate was not difficult for him.

George drew a broader lesson of empowerment from his experience. "To me that is a lesson that there is a consumer-driven health care model where the doctors are competing for patients. And if you have the ability to pick up the phone and reason with a doctor and basically say, 'I'm going to take my business elsewhere,' that can drive down cost, too. And you can benefit from that. But again, that's just one anecdote out of an industry that is 20% of the economy."

A similar anecdote came from Ruby, the high school history teacher and former vintage clothing store owner who I introduced in Chapters 3 and 4. After successful fertility treatment resulted in the birth of her son, she and her husband still had one embryo in storage. "You get a year free," she explained. "It's like cable. Or an adjustable rate mortgage." After the year, the rates go way up. Thousands of dollars in charges began with no reminder. "We called them up and we were like, 'We really thought you would give us a heads up.'" The clinic staff admitted they had no consistent process for notifying patients about costs. They offered to drop most of the charges. From thousands of dollars, Ruby's liability fell to around $60. The experience punctuated the business aspect of clinical services. "We forgot it was like a consumer business thing, and all of a sudden, these people who had been our helpers . . . it was just jarring. It felt like they pulled a fast one." Ruby wasn't especially comfortable with the realization that her trusted partners in a highly emotional and sensitive health care service were operating a business. In that business context, however, Ruby played a vital role in saving her family so much money. "What if I hadn't had the nerve to call?"

At times, negotiating health care costs doesn't work, but it's not for lack of trying. Ralph is a quintessential negotiator introduced in Chapter 4. "If I can negotiate something, I'll try to negotiate it." Now retired, he used to run a family business. Family members and neighbors ask him to negotiate their car prices because he gets good deals. His secret is simple: "You try."

With a thick Boston accent, Ralph told me about trying to negotiate with a doctor after having a lymph node taken out of his neck. He had been billed for two separate operations, done at the same time in the same place by the same physician. "They weren't different operations; they were just different parts of the same operation." The insurance company rejected one of the charges, seeing through the duplicative billing. "From the doctor's point of view, he writes it up in such a way so that he can get a lot more money."

The rest of the bill went to Ralph, a practice known as balance billing. Nearly one-third of privately insured Americans received a surprise bill when their health plan paid less than they had expected.[7] When this happened to Ralph, he challenged the provider. "They didn't care, since this is the way they bill it, and they expect their money."

Worried an unpaid bill would hurt his credit rating, he eventually paid it but didn't feel he should have to. "I told them, 'You've just lost yourself a patient and other references,'" Ralph said angrily but chuckled when I asked how the doctor had responded. "They weren't the least bit distressed. They were just real hard asses about the whole thing, which I couldn't understand because I thought that they were in the wrong." Ralph's efforts yielded the worst-case scenario that prevents most people from even trying to negotiate: the doctor said "no."

Disappointed but not deterred, Ralph still loves to negotiate. "I never mind negotiating on something. If I considered something too high, I will speak to the doctor on it." That's even part of his strategy. "I know most doctors don't like to deal with that, they like to have their business manager or accounting manager talk to people, but I find I get better help, better support, whenever I talk to the doctor, since the doctor doesn't like to be involved. They're less skilled at negotiating, whereas the accounting person is more skilled and they're paid to get more money." He doesn't seem cutthroat, but he pragmatically uses doctors' discomfort in negotiating to his advantage.

IT'S JUST BUSINESS

George, Ruby, and Ralph all recognized their doctor or clinic was operating a business, however high the stakes. Health care providers' ultimate goal may be to help people, cure disease, and ease suffering—rather than maximize profits—but money still changes hands. Whether the form is nonprofit or for-profit, with mission-driven or mercenary intent, these are businesses. In aggregate, the U.S. health care industry accounts for $3.5 trillion each year, gobbling up 18% of America's GDP.[8] Americans pay a growing share of those rising costs, with 46% of privately insured Americans on a high-deductible plan in 2018,[9] up from 25% in 2010.

In that context, it seems reasonable that rules of business would apply. Typically, the value of goods or services relates to the price customers will pay. When that equation is out of whack, the business adjusts to the market or fails. In sectors where the relationship is not clear, people negotiate as a matter of course. What price the market will bear—what people are willing to pay—for goods or services that are unique or hard to value is a matter of trial and error. The seller floats a price; the buyer counters. If they meet somewhere in between, there's a transaction. The market has spoken with a form of negotiation.

Americans expect to negotiate for real estate, cars, and secondhand goods; in these categories, prices are set through the negotiation process. Health care services share some common elements with these categories: costs can be substantial, value is hard to determine, and price is often disconnected from the actual cost of providing the service. Prices vary greatly—across the country or just across town—even for the same service. With no price tags anywhere in sight for most health care services, the category seems ripe for negotiating.

In fact, health care prices *are* set through negotiations—between hospitals, doctors, pharmacies, and health plans.[10] Negotiating leverage accrues to parties with scale, prestige, or specialization. The process is almost always opaque to the consumer.

As consumers take on greater financial responsibility and enter the health care market as customers, they will want to know basic information: What will this cost me? And what options do I have, if any? So far, it's challenging to find easy or satisfactory answers. Health care consumers who pay cash—because they lack insurance, a service they need or want isn't covered, or they have yet to satisfy a deductible—may benefit from trying to negotiate.

Could effective negotiations become a more standard—and easier—cost-saving tactic for American health care consumers? George believes exerting purchasing power and voting with one's feet can lower prices. That's logical and intuitive.

Economics offers a more nuanced picture of the potential impact of negotiating, suggesting that if more of us bargain, initial prices may rise. On the other hand, economists have also shown that in markets with more negotiators, good negotiators representing a small percentage of the total market will do better; sellers will have flexibility to bargain with this minority because they can raise prices for the majority, who are less good at—or just less keen on—negotiating.[11] No matter the study or the context, shrewd negotiators tend to fare well.

But how can Americans—who already avoid negotiating—become better negotiators in a market where negotiating isn't the norm? Not all of us even recognize health care as a market at all. The first step might be to simply recognize that negotiation is a strategy worth trying. Though stories of health care negotiating don't usually look like what happens when you walk into a car dealership or make an offer on a house, negotiations do happen. And they sometimes work.

Based on my consumer interviews and recommendations from negotiation experts, here are five strategies to consider in negotiating health care prices:

1. **Ask if there's an out-of-pocket or cash price, even if you have insurance**

Like Ingrid who asked her doctor "to check the box," Lillian learned to ask about prices explicitly. A nurse still working part-time in her 60s, Lillian had switched to a new Medicare Part D prescription plan that refused to approve the generic estrogen she had been taking for years.

Frustrated with the run-around she experienced appealing the denial, she finally asked the pharmacist, "How much is it if I just pay for it?" The pharmacist—unable to offer the information proactively—responded, "You just asked the magic question!" Gag orders that prevented pharmacists from offering consumers cost-saving tips were common in pharmacy contracts until late 2018 when Congress passed legislation banning the practice.[12]

"I said, 'Just forget it.' I'm not even going to go through arguing with them and getting a prior authorization and then finding out that after I spent all this time, that it's going to be more expensive if I have them pay for it anyways. I might as well just pay for it out of pocket." Lillian paid $19 instead of the $40 copayment she would have paid if insurance approved the prescription. "Now I've gotten smart and I kind of check in on all my meds." Paying out of pocket is often cheaper—sometimes substantially—than using her insurance, which she keeps in case she comes to need a catastrophically expensive medication.

Jason, who earlier said he had never thought of negotiating health care prices, reported trying Lillian's approach in all his health care encounters. He just didn't recognize it as negotiating. "How can I limit the damage?" he asks the front desk staff whenever he goes in for a health care service. "I'll be friendly with them, like, 'Look, I'm trying to make this as cheap as possible. Is there a way that we can reduce the price?'" Jason's insurance deductible is so high that he pays for most health care services out of pocket. By asking about ways to get a better deal, he has learned insurance is not always the cheapest. In Chapter 5, I shared Jason's experience identifying price variation, even at the same location for the same service. As a result, he has learned to always ask about the price, which sometimes unearths a cheaper solution.

2. Put costs on the table with your doctor and other clinicians

Many clinicians embrace ignorance about health care costs. Yet as Chapter 3 shows, therapists can and do discuss costs and sometimes negotiate; others see consistency—and limits—as good for their patients, as well as for their own business interests. Regardless of where they draw the line, the financial aspects of care are explicit which enables therapists to more comfortably and effectively negotiate—or choose not to—than in other parts of medicine.

Heather Ross of Arizona State University advocated that factoring and addressing patient costs is vital to patients' best interests. "Making a decision about a patient's health care without acknowledging cost, and [whether they] can attain what you are directing them to go out into the world and do? To not ask that question and to not craft a medication or a therapeutic plan for a patient that they can reasonably attain in the context of their life economically, that, to me, seems to be ethically problematic."

To help expedite the medical establishment's adaptation to changing economic realities, an important step consumers can take is to ask the questions: What will this cost? Is there a cheaper way for me to get the same benefit? Do I need this? Making cost concerns explicit and seeking to partner with providers in making health care more affordable will help force doctors and other clinicians to prepare themselves for these conversations. Most doctors I know hate to be wrong or unprepared. Ask them questions they don't know enough times, and they're likely to start finding answers.

Sometimes, just asking about costs can open a negotiation. If you ask "how much is this?" at a flea market, merchants commonly follow up the answer with an offer to do better. That second price is often your invitation to negotiate.

Melody, a therapist, described discussing the cost of naturopathy services for what turned out to be premature menopause. "It's just asking the front desk administrator, 'Will my insurance cover this?' And they knew the answers to that. They knew that [my insurance] did not cover services. And they have a set rate for people who are paying out of pocket. They would also work with me. They'd say, 'I think we could probably do a really brief follow-up at a reduced rate.' They were actively trying to keep it accessible." She never asked explicitly for a price break. "Without realizing it, I am saying things as I'm scheduling, 'Well, I don't want to come in too often, because it's expensive.' Not consciously or purposely." By subtly conveying her financial concerns, Melody opened a successful negotiation.

3.   Invest energy in self-advocacy

Much of health care negotiating takes the form of arguing with insurance companies for approval of a service or benefit, or arguing bills after the fact. A *Consumer Reports* survey found that 57% of consumers who had tried to negotiate a medical bill successfully negotiated lower health care bills.[13] Despite deterrents, including time and energy, anxiety or fear of retaliation, and the sometimes "soul-sucking" nature of negotiating, many consumers I interviewed described saving money through self-advocacy.

George and Ruby made a single phone call and knocked hundreds or thousands of dollars off surprise bills. Others, like Angela, a mother of four with an $8,000 deductible, negotiated a payment plan with her hospital to manage her out-of-pocket share of a knee surgery she could not afford outright. She feels she may be paying $50 a month for the rest of her life, but at least the interest-free plan helped when she was not prepared to pay the full amount all at once.

4.   Make the pie bigger

The negotiating stories I heard in my consumer interviews—and the tactics listed earlier—tend to follow the classic zero-sum model. If you let me pay less, you earn less. But there are a few ways everyone can win. For example, if you can, offer to pay cash, and pay it quickly in exchange for a price break. Collecting on medical bills requires an investment by the provider of effort, time, and usually money (paying a vendor to bill and collect and/or paying staff to chase down payments). Time to collect means time without that cash flowing through the operation, and not all bills are ever paid or paid in full. Paying a smaller amount faster with less effort on the provider's part increases value to both parties.

5.   Be nice

Remember the garage-sale sellers who objected to aggressive negotiators? They shut down the sale or stood firm on price when they felt annoyed or disrespected. Follow the American style: be friendly, congenial, jovial. George was ever respectful and cut a third of his bill off. Jason politely engaged provider staff in his quest for lower prices. Explain why you're asking for a break; don't just demand to get a deal like you might at a garage sale. This may not move your doctor's office, and it may not really make the pie bigger in terms of economic value. But, if everyone feels good about the interaction, there is both reputational benefit to the doctor, which could translate into greater loyalty and new patient acquisition, and intrinsic value of a positive experience for everyone.

Health care providers, at least at the institutional level, negotiate with health insurers all the time. They may be less accustomed to negotiating with patients, and some may be downright uncomfortable doing so. But the reality of today's health care dynamics makes financial considerations central for more individuals and their doctors.

Ingrid, who claimed not to negotiate but had done so effectively, did not feel awkward asking for a lower rate. "I feel like everyone sort of gets it," she said. "Like none of us has tons of money." No matter how much money people have, almost no one prefers to pay more than necessary.

Be like Ingrid. Ask.

Just as the Moroccan merchant responded to pressure from his potential buyer, so too might the health care industry respond if consumers band together in search of a better health care bargain.

7

Who's in Charge Here?

How consumers are left alone to navigate their own health care situations

When Margaret's daughter was 6 months old, her husband called while she was at work. A stay-at-home dad, he had taken their baby to her routine well-child checkup. The pediatrician had felt a mass in the baby's abdomen and did not know what it was. That night, the pediatrician biked to Margaret's home—a few towns over—to discuss their options. They could immediately bring the baby to the ER or wait till the morning, when the pediatrician had lined up visits with various specialists.

Margaret and her husband chose the latter and met the next day with the doctors their pediatrician had scheduled. "It was just smooth. They knew what to do. They walked us through it. They held our hands through the process." The pediatrician stayed with them, in a sense, calling to check in as they met different specialists and getting real-time updates from those specialists. "[He] was texting us to just make sure that we were okay and he was offering to connect us to other families that had been through similar experiences. I don't think there are many pediatricians that go above and beyond and have that level of personal service, and making you feel safe, or as safe as possible in a really scary time."

During surgery to remove the baby's mass, the surgeons discovered it had taken over one kidney, which they removed entirely. The tumor turned out to be malignant, but the surgery was a success. The baby needed no further treatment and has had no complications in the seven years since.

Margaret had no such luck when navigating the billing for her own care. In Chapter 2, I described how she found herself stuck in the middle of her health plan and provider, trying to figure out what she owed to resolve a billing issue. "The plan can't really help. You call and they're like, 'The provider needs to resubmit the claim.'" The provider had apparently billed her inconsistently and submitted the claim incorrectly; Margaret had paid the wrong amount through no fault of her own. "I just wanted it to be easy," she said. "I wanted to be able to make one phone call and have it all sorted, but it was just the run-around, between the health plan and then having to call the provider. And you run into people who are not that competent, who don't really understand, and they can't solve your problem, and nor do they seem to really care about solving your problems."

Not everyone has someone watching over their care like a fairy godmother, as Margaret's daughter did. More often—like Margaret with her own billing issue—consumers are left to navigate complex clinical, financial, and administrative situations on their own. Why couldn't the U.S. health system—for all the money Americans collectively spend on it—devote resources to helping people manage care, coverage, and costs?

THE CLINICAL QUARTERBACK

Andrea, a mid-30s mother of three young children, felt alone to navigate in a scary situation. She told me, "I 100% feel I'm my own advocate. My husband's my advocate. We are the quarterbacks. We're in charge of the process."

Andrea first went to the hospital in 2017. She was jaundiced and itching intensely. Doctors discovered the cause: a tumor blocking her bile duct, allowing salts to accumulate and causing her discomfort. Ultimately, they determined the mass was malignant, and she was diagnosed with pancreatic cancer.

Andrea participated in a two-day clinic at the hospital—a top-ranked facility nationally—to consult experts and learn more about her disease and treatment plans. "It was very clear the doctors were not going to spend a lot of time with me on my situation," Andrea said of that first encounter. "They were just going to look at the data and make a decision about the treatment, tell me what the treatment was, ask if I had any questions, and move me out of the office." She had felt rushed, the process impersonal. "It didn't feel like any of the information that we were given was really specific to me. It was more specific to the process. It didn't feel personalized in any way."

That standard package of information didn't feel complete. Andrea and her husband had to figure out the right questions to ask for her specific situation and try to find the right people to talk to. During this process, they met with the oncologist, who explained the options. "The information we were given was basically that it's dealer's choice as to which [chemotherapy] you're put on first, and we didn't like the ambiguity of that guidance."

Believing the surgeon could shed light on the best path forward, Andrea and her husband decided they would not leave the hospital without meeting him. "We just planted ourselves and basically said we'd wait as long as possible so that we could get his perspective."

They got their meeting and trusted the surgeon. Unfortunately, he didn't have a clear answer. "There's just not a lot of research, especially for someone in my particular age group. So, we just had to make a decision based on the information we were given."

Andrea followed the oncologist's recommendation, opting for a less-toxic chemotherapy to start. It didn't work. Her next scan showed that not only hadn't the tumor shrunk but the cancer had actually spread to her liver. Expert advice led Andrea to get herself and the tumor genetic testing, which revealed they should have started her on the other, more aggressive chemotherapy. The doctors did what they thought was best with the information they had. But they clearly did not have—nor seek—information that could have illuminated a more effective treatment for her. Pancreatic cancer survival rates are exceedingly low, and Andrea had wasted time on a drug her doctors could have known was less likely to work.

"We just learned we had to play [quarterback]," Andrea said. "In the past I've always trusted my doctors and kind of did what they said, and this was my first experience with health care where I realized it's not up to them, it's up to me, and I need to figure things out for myself as to how I want to be treated, where I want be treated, and when."

Andrea took charge of her treatment plan, traveling for second and third opinions. She and her family and friends found clinical trials with promising drugs for pancreatic cancer. She felt she couldn't join the trial and risk being put on placebo; with three young children, the stakes were too high. But she was able to get a prescription for the promising drug—paying $15,000 per month out of pocket since insurance wouldn't cover it. That drug worked, shrinking her tumors to the point she could have surgery and effectively putting her into remission.

Andrea was willing and able—especially with her husband's help—to quarterback her care, and it likely saved her life. Though she had the capacity, and the support to do so, she told me, "It's very difficult to be a health care consumer right now. It does feel like there are people who would be very hopeless in navigating health care and getting the right kind of care."

Not everyone has her level of tenacity or resources. "People don't know what questions they're not asking. So it's not like you can figure out what you're doing wrong. A lot of people don't even know that they're doing anything wrong. They're just kind of going through the process. They don't know that there are other options out there."

TAKING A BACK SEAT

Not all consumers could manage Andrea's situation, especially when they're that sick, scared, and vulnerable. Lack of knowledge and competence combine with fear to make quarterbacking one's care difficult for many.

Others face a more fundamental obstacle to actively managing their own health care situations: not all patients *want* to take charge.

"I used to joke that I only ran to the bathroom or if a bear was chasing me," Ruby, a high school history teacher, described her history of physical fitness. As I described in Chapter 2, though she thought of herself as healthy, she spent 17 years smoking a pack of cigarettes a day and not exercising. "When you're a heavy smoker, you don't go to the doctor because you don't want to go and have someone remind you of the horrible stuff you're doing and you don't want to find out anything. So, I avoided going. I made sure I had health insurance and then strenuously avoided going to the doctor for 15 years."

Ruby had grown up accessing care through a health maintenance organization (HMO), where you just didn't shop or even focus on the individual doctor. "You just went to whomever they thought could give you the care. I just didn't understand the idea of picking a doctor."

When Ruby started teaching, she signed up for health insurance and had to pick a primary care physician (PCP), but she was "terrified of bureaucracy and of having to make phone calls in grown-up ways. . . . I basically just opened the big book and I started calling. The first person who said they had room, that was who I went with. And I then, of course, never saw that person ever. Never went in for a single appointment. Educated consumer, not so much."

In her first year of teaching, Ruby got pneumonia. "I was supposed to go to my primary care physician, but I didn't actually know who that was, because remember, I just opened the book, signed up, and then I didn't remember. And then I was too scared to call Blue Cross Blue Shield to find out who it was, so I didn't." She sought out a family friend—a physician—who confirmed Ruby had pneumonia and wrote her a prescription. "I didn't go to see a doctor again for 12 years, until I started dating my husband."

Luckily, Ruby married someone who is keenly attentive to health care needs and decisions. "I don't manage our health care at all. My husband does all of it. . . . He's kind of hypochondriacal. He probably wouldn't say that; he would say he's concerned appropriately." Without him, how would Ruby navigate her health care needs since she clearly has no interest in doing so?

Ruby's health system avoidance may be extreme but it is representative of consumers who don't want to drive their health care lives. There could be myriad reasons for lack of consumer engagement: discomfort with bureaucracy, fear of bad health care news, or abundant trust in professionals. Some consumers are simply uninterested in health care; if they're lucky, they need it infrequently and can afford not to focus on it.

Curtis, a businessperson based in San Francisco's Bay Area, had seen ample evidence of consumer apathy. His firm had invested in a company that originally provided hospitals with patient portals—secure websites to provide patients access to information about their medical care. For a time, the federal government offered financial incentives to encourage hospitals to provide these online tools, but the availability of tools did not drive consumer adoption.

"I don't think consumers are pounding on the table for hospitals to have a patient portal," Curtis explained. "The hospitals were implementing it because they were getting money from the government to do it." These portals are more complicated than they look, requiring technology to stitch together disparate back-end systems and data sources and translate that data into consumer-accessible formats. The portals didn't always work well, but that may not have mattered. "It's not like your Bank of America website going down, [where] everybody's going to hear about it right away." The more important finding from those early days was that consumers just didn't use them. By 2017, nearly all hospitals offered patient portals, but nearly two-thirds reported fewer than 25% of patients using them.[1]

Curtis had assumed patient portals were a key component of the consumerization of health care. Making patients' own medical records available to them could provide insight into their visits, lab tests, and procedures over time. They could enable consumers to understand their health status and make data-driven health care decisions. Just as you might see at a glance how your retirement account is performing, he thought consumers would want to "slice and dice it six different ways and see what it looks like over time." But consumer demand was not there for this level of insight and the control it could allow.

Information asymmetry is one of the major obstacles cited to health care consumerism because consumers are on unequal footing with doctors in decision-making processes. Yet presented with opportunities to access more information, most consumers did not use the available information. Thus, information asymmetry is not just a function of lack of clinical education and training among consumers; it reflects limited consumer will. It's hard enough for consumers to actively manage their health, harder still if they don't use the data available to them.

AN ADMINISTRATIVE VORTEX

Curtis's perspective on the value of these kinds of tools was informed not just by his professional experience but by an unfortunate clinical encounter as well. He had sat by his son's intensive care unit bedside for two weeks after a traumatic spinal cord injury. Curtis vividly remembered the harrowing early moments when his son was rushed into the ICU. Somebody from the hospital's finance department prompted him to sign a form committing to take personal financial responsibility for anything his health plan wouldn't cover. "That form gets shoved at you when your child is getting prepped [for] surgery to operate on his broken neck. If I would have said 'no,' would they have wheeled him out of there or given him to some undergrad biology student to work on? I have no idea. What do you do in that case? You sign what they put in front of you." Economists point to moments like these, correctly, to illustrate the limitations of consumer power in health care decisions. Curtis had no choice.

When the hospital and the health plan reached an impasse on $250,000 of an almost $1 million bill from that encounter, the hospital was within its rights to send Curtis the bill, except Curtis never received a bill and learned of his liability only when he began getting collections notices.

"That issue took a year and a half to get resolved." But it did get resolved because of Curtis's thoroughness and perseverance. Curtis had kept close watch on his son's care and was well versed in what had transpired. He used that knowledge when he found himself stuck between the hospital and the health plan.

"It was a huge back and forth, and I was in the middle." Curtis plotted all the invoices on a spreadsheet and analyzed each line item. Some charges had been paid in full, some for pennies on the dollar, and some had not been paid at all, including the neck surgery itself. Where the plan had paid nothing, or nothing reasonable, Curtis pushed back.

It wasn't easy. "You get the run-around a lot at the insurance companies and finally they assigned a person to me, to help figure this out. And now you explain the same thing to ten different people and then finally, you get the one person who can help solve the problem."

The bureaucratic vortex Curtis found himself in was in effect on the hospital side too; it took an in-person interaction with the neurosurgeon for Curtis to get a return call. That worked. Eventually, the quarter-million-dollar bill was resolved, with Curtis paying almost none of it.

Curtis's son regained a remarkable amount of mobility, though he may never heal fully. And Curtis avoided a financial disaster. But he had to take extraordinary measures to do so. He had sophisticated financial analysis and management skills and the diligence and determination to follow every line item through the process to the end.

Consumers shouldn't need Curtis's level of financial competence to navigate their bills. Health plans and hospitals should recognize the humans in the middle of their negotiations and shield consumers from unreasonable expense and stress. It all worked out in the end, but ensuring resolution should be a corporate responsibility, not just an extreme consumer burden.

FIGHTING FOR BREATH

Austin, whose story appears in Chapter 3, found himself forced to navigate his own health benefits. His new job—a public service role with a government agency—wasn't going to cover his allergy medication. "They were telling me that was a preexisting condition, so they wouldn't treat it," he said. "But I needed [treatment] to exist." Having moved to a new city, his allergies were flaring, triggering asthma. He couldn't breathe.

A recent college graduate working for extremely low wages, he could not afford to buy the medications on his own. He couldn't believe the agency hiring him, not a third-party insurer, was denying his access to medication. (An insurer would not have been allowed to withhold treatment for a preexisting condition under the Affordable Care Act.) "They were putting me in a position where, in order to do the job that they were asking me to do, my health was at risk, because asthma is very serious. My ability to do pretty much anything is predicated on my ability to breathe."

Austin advocated for himself vociferously, stubbornly sticking with the fight against this policy. "I just kept going back and forth with people and then getting moved up to another manager or something, because I wouldn't get off the phone and I don't think they were allowed to hang up on me. I kept arguing and arguing and talking to people. Eventually, someone listened when I was talking about. 'Your time is a lot more valuable and I'm not going to stop tying up the lines here for people.'" Austin's persistence paid off. "I ended up solving it by being on the phone with them for hours and hours until it was cost effective for them to decide to get me off the phone." After probably eight total hours on the phone, he did get his medications covered.

Now he could breathe, but he wasn't happy about the process. "It's incredibly frustrating that you need to waste a lot of time justifying your right to your own health with people in order to have insurance providers, or in this case, government health coverage providers, give the things that they should be giving."

As a white male, Austin felt comfortable—and even responsible for—holding his employer accountable. He viewed the advocacy for his medication coverage as bigger than himself, a form of navigation on behalf of others because many people "don't grow up learning you complain until you get your way, and who don't have the kind of privilege that gets people to respect them and continue to listen." Austin felt he could fight for the right thing because he was confident, competent, and entitled to get what he knew he deserved. He did not think he alone deserved it and recognized that because he could fight for it, he should—on behalf of consumers who may not feel they could advocate for themselves or have a chance of resolving the situation in their favor.

EASING CONSUMERS' BURDENS

Should consumers bear the burden of navigating their own health care, clinically as in Andrea's case or administratively as in Margaret's, Curtis's, or Austin's?

In a perfect world, someone would be assigned to help each consumer navigate the system during the most complex situations and be on call for annoying snafus resulting from more routine care. Such a person would not only be expert in the nuances and crevices of health care bureaucracies; he or she would also be extraordinarily resilient, using knowledge to track down the path to meeting the consumer's specific needs. The consumer's ideal partner would be someone to take charge when they cannot, to guide or inform those who prefer to drive their own decisions, or to answer questions no matter how mundane or knotty. Such a person to accompany consumers through their health care lives could work for any number of health care entities—the primary care doctor's office, the hospital, or the health plan. Each has a stake, theoretically, in the consumer's smooth navigation of the system and should have the requisite perspective and knowledge to help.

In reality, these people may only exist in the form of case or care managers for the most acute—as in expensive—health plan members, or the most vulnerable, complex, and often indigent hospital or clinic patients. Most consumers get no support at all.

For example, despite the severity of Curtis's son's injuries, they got very little help to manage his recovery. After two weeks in intensive care, Curtis's son spent six weeks in a rehabilitation hospital. He was still severely injured when he was discharged. "There was a whole regimen that we had to follow at home to make sure he didn't take a backward step. I'm a pretty educated person and I'm pretty organized, and I found this stuff to be really complicated."

Curtis thought about others who might be in this situation. How would less-organized people fare? "There's a really good chance that you could screw it up." Curtis's son needed attention and different medications throughout the day, following a strict schedule to avoid bedsores or other complications. Curtis was shocked that they got essentially no instructions or support upon discharge from the rehabilitation hospital, not even a checklist. "We're scrambling to write the notes to figure this out," he recalled. People do typically get discharge instructions when leaving the hospital or rehab facility, but obviously in Curtis's case and likely many others, they were insufficient or missing altogether. It can be hard to absorb these instructions when leaving the hospital and harder still to implement complex routines on their own at home.

Ironically, through his work, Curtis knew intimately that solutions could exist to enable better follow-up care. "We were at a hospital that sits right smack dab in the middle of Silicon Valley and the technology's out there to do this," he reflected. "This is not new tech but it's not being applied to this area. And that just astounded me."

Instead of writing notes to track the details of his son's complex care, "I'm thinking there should be a website I go to and somebody should send me a text message every day saying . . . 'Hey, just want to make sure that you did these three things' and they should do that every day for the first three weeks that they're back at home."

"But you didn't see any of that?" I asked.

"No, not at all."

Curtis contrasted the lack of a solid handoff from rehab with the service he gets for his car, where the follow-up is phenomenal. "When I'm within 2,000 miles of having to take it in for the maintenance, I'm getting the emails on it, they're trying to upsell me on different things or let me know about new models that come out. But that same thing for my son? Nothing. It's crazy." The car dealership sees financial value in maintaining a good relationship with Curtis; he'll pay for service and buy his next car there, and he might recommend others do the same.

But the acute-care hospital and rehab facilities that treated his son do not seem to recognize financial or other value in delighting consumers, even though many hospitals do compete for patient volume even as they increasingly face financial penalties when patients return to the hospital too soon after being discharged. Hospitals that do care could learn some tactics from Curtis's car dealer.

While waiting for entrepreneurs to create solutions to fill the void Curtis described, and for hospital and health plans to implement new tools, what can consumers do to get through the vast and twisty health care maze?

There are no easy answers. Health care won't simplify itself anytime soon. Structural changes that could improve consumer support would likely require investment in new staff—and retraining existing staff—which would add costs to an already-bloated system. Health care leaders would need to conjure both imagination and conviction in the business value of such consumer support. Until those factors come together, or until health care organizations resolve the underlying system complexity, consumers need to take charge of their health care.

Even in a more perfect health care world, there is probably no getting around the need for consumers to navigate the health care world. Here are a few approaches to keep in mind when you find yourself in a complex health care situation.

1.   Seek an advocate, point of contact, or other kind of helper

Ask your doctor's office, hospital, or health plan if they can provide you with a single point of contact to help you navigate billing or clinical issues, likely to be different people for each type of issue. Many health care insiders I know think the answer is simple: your PCP is your point of contact. That may be true in theory, but most PCPs are so busy that it can be hard to reach them directly. Ask whom you should call if your doctor cannot help or doesn't call you back.

If you started a small business, your bank would probably assign someone to be your account manager, the person to call if you have questions or need help, and, of course, sell you more banking services. If you organize your kid's birthday party at a facility like an indoor amusement or trampoline park or arcade, the facility would probably assign a host at least on the day of the party—if not beforehand to help plan the event—to make sure everything goes smoothly.

Such an account management or host model is sorely lacking in health care. Hospitals typically have financial counselors and care managers, health plans have customer service representatives, and there's always an escalation point. If they deem your case complex enough, they might assign someone to help you. If not, try asking if they can or at least whom to speak to directly about your issue. Get the person's name and direct phone number. Be persistent. Ask for a time to speak. Ask when to expect they can get back to you, and follow up if they do not.

2.   Escalate

When the frontline staff person cannot or will not help you, press on. Somewhere in every organization is someone with the power to negotiate, reverse a decision, or modify a bill. If you hear "We don't negotiate" or "I can't help you," you may be talking to the wrong person. After you've escalated and you hear that, at least you know you've pushed your case as far as you can.

Noah, a graduate student who bought individual insurance, got knocked off his health plan after open enrollment had ended. "I had to do what they called an escalation." It took 8 or 10 hours on the phone with his state's insurance marketplace, "with various people and promises of being called back to complete my application. There was very little consistency and I waited for a lot of phone calls back that didn't come. And then eventually, finally, I talked to one guy who just said, 'Oh, no this is very simple. Here's what we need to do. Here's what you're eligible for based on your income. Here's what the copays will be.' And actually explained the whole system to me." It worked out for Noah but not without immense frustration over customer service inconsistency and incompetence.

Austin stayed on the phone to resolve his medication coverage dispute until he found someone with the authority to resolve the issue. He felt perfectly empowered to escalate, moving up the hierarchy. He felt confident in his position. Emboldened by the obvious injustice he felt he was suffering by not being able to get his asthma medicine, and his own sense of white-male privilege, he sought out authority whom he correctly assumed would recognize the merits of his argument.

Not everyone feels so entitled to resolution. Studies show that although vulnerable or disadvantaged consumers often experience worse customer service,[2] they are less likely to complain when dissatisfied with a shopping experience.[3,4] That needs to change. Disparities, and resulting consumer passivity in seeking remedies, have accumulated over centuries. Yet if all health care consumers felt entitled to resolution—and consistently escalated until receiving it—health care organizations would have to respond by raising their level of customer support, especially for vulnerable consumers who need it most.

Consumers are not necessarily entitled to a specific, preferred outcome, but everyone should feel entitled to lay out their case and try to get a fair hearing. If something doesn't feel right—logical, fair, consistent—it is completely reasonable to want to make sure the person on the other end of your complaint has the authority to decide not to help you. Once, when a deal I was trying to negotiate stalled at an unsatisfactory point, I asked the person I was negotiating with to confirm that for her large organization sticking to their terms was more important than closing a deal. She paused and reiterated the terms on the table, effectively conveying, "Take it or leave it." I wasn't happy with the outcome, but at least I could be sure there was no better resolution available.

When you reach the end of the line with no resolution, and you aren't ready to give up, there can be other ways to escalate, such as taking your case to authorities, if there are consumer protection agencies governing the dispute. Or you can take it public. For example, Angela, a mother of four described in the Introduction, was facing a billing dispute when we spoke. She had taken one of her children to an urgent-care center for a strep test and received a bill as if she had gone to the emergency room. Angry over what she felt was false advertising, Angela was fighting the bill, so far unsuccessfully. She sought advice from health care experts she knew and planned to escalate publicly to ensure oversight of the misleading practice. "I'll write a letter to the paper. I'll call up a news station and say, 'You've got to be reporting on this because this is ridiculous.'"

To take this approach, you must be sure your case is sympathetic and clear. If a bureaucracy is depriving you of care, or charging you unfairly, the public may identify with you. Even a simple letter to the editor of the local paper can help you get some attention. But if there's gray area—where there's a clear rule posted or the average person might not take your side— it might be time to cut your losses and accept the answer.

3. Advocate

As much as consumers want to be supported in their health care encounters, consumer stories repeatedly show the need for self-advocacy.

After a traumatic accident while riding her bicycle, Megan needed extensive oral surgery. Her jaw had to be wired shut, and she survived on a liquid diet. "They were trying to make sure that your teeth line up at the end of it all. If it heals in the wrong place, they have to re-break your jaw."

At that critical moment, "I did not feel like the person who was doing my follow-up was listening to me when I was telling him that my jaw wasn't lining up." She consulted a dentist who listened and validated that her teeth were not matching up, and told her, "You should talk to them soon, before it's too late and your jaw freezes in the wrong place."

Megan got a second opinion and switched to a new doctor. He adjusted the alignment of her teeth without needing to re-fracture her jaw. If she hadn't spoken up when she did, she probably would have needed more surgery.

Similarly, Gregg, who appears in Chapters 5 and 6, did his homework and stood up for himself. "I am a firm believer in being proactive," Gregg had learned as the primary caretaker for a dying parent. "I had a lot of experience dealing with doctors, who were very fine physicians. But I did realize that there was a lot of negotiating that needed to be done and that the squeaky wheel gets the oil, or whatever the phrase is."

Gregg applied this lesson to his own health care needs. He investigated whether a vitamin D deficiency might be causing a minor chronic condition. "My doctor had no inkling of suggesting that I get checked. I told him I wanted to have it checked." Gregg's hunch was right; he did have low vitamin D levels—a solvable problem. Through his own efforts, he found a possible solution on his own. Three months of high-dose vitamin D resolved a condition he'd lived with for 20 years. "If I hadn't taken the initiative, I would still be suffering from that chronic condition, and it probably would've gotten a lot worse."

4.   Come prepared

Consumers who stay on top of their health care needs and situations are better prepared to navigate and self-advocate. "When you're in the driver's seat and you get to decide what kind of treatment you want," Eliza said, "you're really in that position of deciding what's best for you."

Though just in her 20s, Eliza had had several experiences that required she navigate her own health care journey, from billing mistakes to being given the wrong treatment. Responsible by nature, these experiences made her more vigilant and proactive about her health care. She was also raised on her mother's philosophy: "You take health care into your own hands." To Eliza, that meant trying to understand her insurance and the services being recommended or performed, and communicating as much information as she could to her physicians to make sure they can help as much as possible. "The more information I can arm myself with, the better, so that I know, when I am paying for the treatment that it makes sense."

In Eliza's view, health care involves a series of decisions, which the consumer can't always see, so you have to "make sure that you stay on top of things. If you don't feel well, you go to the doctor. You research what it is you have. You ask a lot of questions. You make sure that you're taking whatever it is that you need to take." Of course, there's a lot of misleading evidence online too, so it helps to check the source and lean on expert consensus rather than individual anecdotes.

5.   Take notes

You may find yourself alone in the health care maze. Your situation may not rise to the level that requires extra attention from your health plan or hospital, so you may not have access to dedicated help. Even if you get help, you might still need to advocate for yourself.

In these instances, you are likely to fare better at navigating and advocating for yourself if you take notes—literally. In my interviews, the people who had found resolution to their challenges were organized and thorough. They kept detailed notes and used those records as the basis for their self-advocacy. These people exerted enormous effort to get what they needed—resolution of a billing problem or clinical care that suited one's own unique case. They were all capable and competent, but above all, they were persistent. Having documentation of your experience makes it easier to persist; the facts on your side won't always get you the resolution you want, but it helps. Having those facts documented can mean a lot less hassle for you.

6.   Vote with your feet

It shouldn't have to be so hard to navigate the health care system, especially when you are sick or stressed out about your health or your finances.

New kinds of health care providers are emerging, and switching to one might be the easiest way to find accompaniment on your health care journey.

A movement to redesign primary care and reimagine health care delivery is afoot. Start-up practices may offer more modern approaches to ease consumer burdens for scheduling, convenient hours, billing and payments, and following up with specialists.

Concierge practices typically serve fewer patients and operate outside of the insurance system. Though patients pay out of pocket, often a flat fee, they typically get round-the-clock access—or at least more access—to their doctor. Without worrying about filing insurance claims and optimizing billing codes, doctors in these practices are usually willing to consult by phone, text, and email. Because these practices do not need to employ whole billing departments to interface with insurers, they can invest in consumer support.

Akin to concierge practices, direct primary care providers also operate outside of health insurance and offer access to the primary care doctor for a typically more modest monthly fee. While still relatively uncommon, this approach is growing rapidly, with the number of direct primary care patients tripling between 2015 and 2017.[5]

These types of practices are not always accessible and can be costly, but they are on the rise. Joining one, if it's an option, may be the loudest signal a consumer can send about the need for the traditional health care system to improve consumer support.

AN EDUCATED CONSUMER

Consumers must often navigate their health care issues on their own. Too often, it seems to be no one's job to help the consumer resolve issues large and small. In other businesses with expensive services, staff are assigned to help the customer navigate. Not so for most health care consumers. I remember once scouring my health plan ID card looking for a basic customer service phone number, and then digging into the plan website, to no avail. "I guess they don't want phone calls," I remember thinking.

With health care costs rising and immense pressure to slow those cost increases, it is unlikely health plans and providers will introduce a new service layer with costly additional staff. But they could create channels of communication for consumers navigating health insurance and health services.

Some of the biggest frustrations I have heard from consumers is getting the run-around—being stuck between a health plan and provider as they fight out the bill—and not knowing even where to begin when navigating the health care system. Health care organizations should create clear pathways for inquiries, escalation, and more intensive help—and let consumers self-identify for the level of service they need or want. They should train staff for and create a culture of accountability and a bias toward resolution. As consumers feel accompanied rather than alone to shoulder health care navigation burdens, they will capture greater value and build trust in health care institutions.

Consumers should request those kinds of supports. It requires effort to create a drumbeat for better service and to refuse to tolerate being stuck in between health care behemoths. Ultimately, investing such energy may be the most effective path to systemic change in how consumers are treated. Until such changes become reality, consumers may need to be their own champions, reminding the health system that "an educated consumer is our best customer."[6]

8

Listen!

Why consumers' own voices are often overlooked and what we lose as a result

---

Amanda didn't go to the hospital at first. A young professional with a long history of chronic stomach pains that came and went—at times intense enough to keep her from working or going out with friends—she did not want to repeat her last health care encounter. In that instance, her stomach pains were more intense than she had ever experienced. Because she worked for a health policy think tank, she tried to be responsible in how she sought care. It was the middle of the day, and after carefully studying her health plan's website to understand what she was "supposed to do," she drove herself to a plan-operated urgent-care clinic, crying on the way from severe pain. Her reward for avoiding expensive emergency room care should have been a $75 charge for the visit.

The physician assistant (PA) who examined her ordered several tests for things Amanda knew were not problems because she had just had a physical. Still, the PA insisted. "I was writhing in pain on the table. I wasn't going to fight tooth and nail to skip these tests, but I made it very clear that it was not necessary and that I did not want to do them." The test results came back normal, as Amanda had expected.

"After taking a lot of tests, which I later learned were not the right tests, they dismissed me and the diagnosis was like 'undiagnosable pain.' It was a

119

German word that is actually a diagnosis for female pain that cannot be diagnosed." Amanda may have been diagnosed with *mittelschmerz*, a medical term for mid-menstrual-cycle pain that is not necessarily treatable. She left with what felt like a pat on the head and what turned out to be a $700 bill. "Nothing came of that whole visit."

Amanda never went to the doctor during the next episode. "I cried through it," she admitted. "I chose not to go to the ER because that initial trip had cost me hundreds of dollars, and [the pain] did go away on its own after an eight-hour episode that first time."

The cost of that prior experience was only part of her decision to stay home the second time. "There's something almost embarrassing or humiliating about going to the hospital and being discharged with whatever this diagnosis was that they gave me. Even if there was a funny name for it. It still makes you feel like you shouldn't have gone in, and you did something wrong by coming in. I think all of those emotional factors played into me choosing not to go the next time."

A month later came a third acute episode. "After seven hours of waiting it out I couldn't take it anymore." It was 4:00 A.M. and the closest hospital was not associated with her health plan. She couldn't recall exactly how she figured out that in an emergency, her insurance would have to cover the cost. "Once I realized I was one block from potential help, I decided to go." After scans and more tests, she got her diagnosis—appendicitis—and went promptly to the operating room for emergency surgery to remove her appendix. She stayed overnight and had round-the-clock care until she was sent home, approximately 30 hours after she had arrived. "I just saw the dollar signs flashing before my eyes." Ironically, her bill was about $500, less than the two-hour visit to the nonemergency clinic she had visited initially.

MISSED DIAGNOSIS

Amanda's experience is not especially unusual. Diagnostic errors occur in nearly 20% of appendicitis cases;[1] in one study, the odds of a missed appendicitis diagnosis were 30% greater among women than men.*

Almost any way you calculate diagnostic errors—including missed, delayed, or incorrect diagnoses—they are frighteningly common. An estimated 12 million people who seek outpatient care in the United States

---

* In this study, the odds of a false positive were even greater: 130% greater for women than men. Both measures suggest differences in diagnosis of women compared to men.

experience some form of diagnostic error,[2] and another analysis suggests 1 million people are harmed in the United States each year as a result.[3] The diagnostic error rate can be as high as 50%, depending on diagnosis.[4] For example, in one study, 40% of lung cancer cases had missed diagnostic opportunities, which prolonged time to diagnosis by nearly four months.[5] Among individuals with an ultimate diagnosis of bipolar disorder, at least one-third waited 10 years or more for the correct diagnosis.[6]

In *When Doctors Don't Listen*,[7] Drs. Leana Wen and Joshua Kosowsky describe processes that lead to missed diagnoses—such as "diagnostic momentum" in which doctors unduly focus on a colleague's suggestion to the exclusion of other potential diagnoses, overemphasizing particular symptoms, or focusing too quickly on too narrow a set of possibilities. Constrained by time, experience, and pattern recognition, as well as sometimes imperfect patient reporting, doctors can have the best intentions and still miss things.

Missed diagnoses are a bigger problem for women. Women wait longer than men for treatment of abdominal pain in the emergency room (ER) and are less often prescribed painkillers for such pain[8] despite evidence that women are more likely to experience pain than men[9,10] and at greater intensity.[11] Even after heart surgery, women received more sedatives and fewer painkillers,[12] and were more likely to be prescribed psychotropic drugs[13]—at times inappropriately—than men. Women are also more likely to be diagnosed with mental health conditions when they present with chronic pain.[14]

A heart-wrenching essay[15] in *The Atlantic* detailed one woman's experience of being ignored in the ER by a doctor so confident in his initial diagnosis he never checked her CT scan. The woman survived but waited nearly 15 hours in excruciating pain for another doctor to find that the scan showed a mass on her ovary and to get her the care she had needed on arrival.

In another essay, an African American author described a lifetime of infuriating medical treatment[16]—or lack thereof. At age 12, her pain from a softball-sized ovarian cyst was long ignored, putting her life at risk. Years later, she was again ignored after spinal surgery, despite worsening pain, until she fainted in an elevator at the doctor's office and finally got the surgeon's attention. Another woman's cervical cancer diagnosis—and recognition of recurrence—was delayed by doctors who discounted her symptoms.[17] Those delays may have cost her life.

These stories piercingly illustrate the harm gender and racial bias can cause in health care diagnosis and treatment, as does a *New England Journal of Medicine* study that showed women were more likely than men to be sent home from the hospital in the middle of a heart attack, as were nonwhites versus whites.[18] Worse, failure to admit people to the hospital was associated with higher mortality. Bluntly, people sent home during a heart attack were more likely to die.

It is not clear whether insidious gender bias directly or subtly influenced Amanda's treatment at the urgent-care center. Whether negligence or ingrained bias, ignoring patients' voices negatively impacts health care quality, costs, and patients' trust in the system.

Overlooking women's health concerns is a longstanding medical tradition. The concept of hysteria—which explained a wide range of women's health complaints for centuries—is derived from the Greek word for "womb." The ancient Greeks were "positively obsessed with the womb"[19] and blamed it for a wide range of physical ailments in women, including death. Ancient Egyptians likewise attributed aches, pains, and all manner of psychological problems to "wandering wombs";[20] a starved or dislodged uterus was thought to wreak havoc as it moved about the body. In the 1700s, the medical field began recognizing psychological sources rather than physical ones for symptoms of hysteria, and Freud later linked these issues to the brains of both sexes. Hysteria came off the American Psychiatric Association's diagnostic menu only in the 1950s, and "hysterical neurosis" remained in the *Diagnostic and Statistical Manual of Mental Disorders*—the authoritative guide for psychiatric diseases—until 1980.[21]

BUREAUCRATIC SEXISM

Gender bias was part of the problem for Ingrid, a California public-school teacher. Logical and straightforward, she is enmeshed in issues of race and social justice as a white elementary school teacher of mostly students of color.

Ingrid signed up for Kaiser-Permanente insurance when she started her first Bay Area teaching job in 2002. It wasn't the only option, but it was the only free one. People told her the care through Kaiser would be excellent unless "you have a special problem and you'd have to fight for care if you have a problem."

Kaiser is a comprehensive, closed health care system; they offer virtually any service a patient could need and try not to refer patients to non-Kaiser doctors because they have the full spectrum of specialists on staff. If you're not happy with the available doctors, Ingrid was told, it can be hard to get permission to go outside that system.

Nonetheless, Kaiser appealed to Ingrid philosophically. "I'm drawn to the idea of best practices. I believe Kaiser thinks about issues and finds best practices. I believe with Blue Cross, when you go to your individual doctor you're on your own. I like the idea of consensus." Ingrid assumed physicians who work for Kaiser, an integrated organization, must collaborate and decide together on the best approaches. She was not even 30 years old and healthy, earning a starting teacher's salary. She went with Kaiser then, and all these years later deemed it to have been "good enough."

After having two children in her 40s, Ingrid started to develop health problems. "I noticed the other mothers were getting better and I was still bloated and looking eight months pregnant." She was suffering from non-specific digestive issues but could not get a diagnosis.

Her own primary care doctor seemed harried and tired, a new mother herself whose baby didn't sleep. "She spent three years telling me there's nothing wrong with me and I just need more sleep. I felt like there was some truth to that" but also that the doctor's own experience might be coloring her assessment. Ingrid's postpartum visits felt rushed, and she felt uninteresting to the doctor, whose focus areas listed on the website included maternal and child health care in the developing world. "So, I picked another doctor and she listened to me and right away said, 'We'll get you a GI doctor and get this sorted out.' And she did."

When Ingrid switched teaching jobs not long before we spoke, she contemplated paying more for a non-Kaiser plan. "I'm starting to get a few [health] issues. And sure enough, it's been hard to advocate for myself. I've managed to get them addressed but it's just what people said. You have to break through your provider—their initial resistance at offering you any referral. . . . I kept bringing things up and I felt they told me it was fine. It took three years before anyone listened to me about my digestion issues."

Ingrid attributed her experience to "bureaucratic sexism." Even though her doctor was female—and a new mother at that—Ingrid felt the broader medical system was entrenched in gender bias, with which her feeling of being dismissed was intertwined. "Mothers don't always advocate for ourselves. We put ourselves last." When Ingrid felt her concerns were not being taken seriously, she experienced it as misogyny. "Kaiser needs to do something about really listening to people. They need education on gender issues." Even in a well-regarded health system like Kaiser, individual doctors gave Ingrid the sense that her concerns were not important, let alone real. Ingrid was left on her own to push for the care she needed.

THE COST OF BEING IGNORED

How many doctor visits were wasted while Amanda and Ingrid sought concrete diagnoses for their nonspecific problems? And at what cost—to themselves and to the system?

Though it is difficult to calculate direct costs associated with diagnostic errors, estimates of the annual cost of outright medical errors range from $1 billion[22] to nearly $20 billion.[23,24] Medical error is calculated to be the third-leading cause of death, after heart disease and cancer.[25] Tangibly, the costs are high.

Intangible costs also shape consumer engagement with the health care system. The women I interviewed articulated mistrust, resignation, and avoidance resulting from bad experiences in which they had not felt heard. These feelings diminished their subsequent willingness to even try to get the care they needed. When they did finally seek care, their needs were more likely to be acute and more costly to treat.

Amanda's frustration with her quest for a diagnosis for her chronic stomach pain had "created this whole emotional challenge or tension between me and my trust in the health system. It feels like I've never had a breakthrough in this discovery process, and so I've sort of given up, which means I just don't really go. I've stopped trying to get to the bottom of it." Without a concrete diagnosis, sometimes Amanda felt clinicians were not interested in her case. "There's nothing really fascinating medically about what's going on, unless there is some crazy thing at the heart of all my woes."

Without capturing a doctor's attention, patient voices—and the value they bring to diagnosis and treatment—can be lost. "I feel like I am the one who knows the situation better than anyone else," Amanda expressed. "No doctor's been able to give me any information about what biologically is going on."

THE POWER OF LISTENING

While many consumers describe not feeling heard, some doctors do care a lot about listening—and some even teach about it. Suzanne Koven, MD, takes a novel approach to listening, through the art of storytelling in medicine.

"There's just nothing more therapeutic, and nothing more essential to developing an effective, trusting relationship with a health care giver than having your story listened to, and specifically listened to in the way you want to tell it, not being interrupted, not being told to speed over the parts that the caregiver doesn't want to hear," Koven told me. A primary care doctor and inaugural writer-in-residence at Massachusetts General Hospital, she facilitates literature and poetry discussion groups with hospital staff, clinicians, and trainees. "Stories remind us of our common humanity, and automatically increase our empathy," she said. "If you know someone's story, it's really hard not to empathize with them."

The power of stories in medicine is clear. Stories build trust and enable bonding between patients and providers. "With somebody you trust, you're going to be more forthcoming, and provide information that's going to be helpful in planning your care. There's something about feeling that you are closely accompanied on this particular journey . . . by somebody who's medically knowledgeable but who also really cares about you."

Hearing a more complete version of patient stories improves doctors' diagnostic capabilities. "If you don't hear the full story with all its contradiction and nuance, it narrows the scope," Koven explained. "You want to have as large an array of possibilities as you can to consider. If you're listening to a story in a very narrow way, then your list of possibilities is going to be more limited. It has very real consequences." The patient's story, which doctors can only get comprehensively by building trust and listening well, is important diagnostically. It's not just "mushy, squishy stuff."

Koven directly experienced the tangible value of listening after an injury that required surgery on her arm. Upon returning to work, the occupational health nurse required her to have twice as much time as normal for her typical tasks. That accommodation doubled her normal 15- and 30-minute visits. "I was much more relaxed, and because I was more relaxed, the patient was more relaxed." Koven also learned "there was something about minute 17 when things seem to happen." The real reason for someone's visit would emerge, or the patient would offer a meaningful insight relevant to the diagnosis. The opportunity to listen gave Koven a deeper understanding and truer picture of patients' needs.

Doctors tell me they often race through busy appointment schedules, prescribing medications, tests, or referrals to specialists before moving on to the next patient; it can be the easiest way to stay on schedule in the typical rapid-fire pace of clinical care. Yet, in this temporarily slower pace, Koven was better able to learn the root causes of someone's primary complaint. She noted that stress or loneliness might sometimes be the real reason for patients' visits, which no test or prescription could solve. "I realized I was costing the health care system a lot less money, because 15 minutes of my time is a lot cheaper than an endoscopy." Listening has immense power for the individuals involved and positive implications for the system as a whole.

THE PROMISE OF SHARED DECISION-MAKING

Listening to patients allows another practice proven to improve patient satisfaction and lower health care costs: shared decision-making. The concept is simple: involve patients in their health care decisions. It is so simple that it's hard to believe we need a term for it, let alone extensive research to prove its merits.

But shared decision-making has not been the historical norm in health care. The concept arose in the early 1970s against a backdrop of paternalistic medical culture in which doctors decided treatments for patients. Doctors were charged with doing no harm and assumed to know best. Emerging values of equal rights, pursuit of personal fulfillment, and questioning authority began to spill over into medicine. Out of ethical considerations for patients' freedom and dignity, Robert Veatch, a Georgetown professor and a pioneer of biomedical ethics,[26] argued for sharing decision-making with patients as a means of ensuring all people's right to health care.[27]

At the root of shared decision-making is the reality that even doctors don't always know the answer. Often, there isn't a clear, right answer. Absent clear evidence—and sometimes despite it—clinicians often rely on "clinical gestalt,"[28] essentially pattern recognition used to make decisions with imperfect information. Informed by experience, these shortcuts simplify complex decision-making but also introduce cognitive biases that can lead to errors.[29,30] That said, physician judgment may outperform standard decision pathways,[31] and Drs. Wen and Kosowsky strenuously argue against "cookbook medicine" that diminishes the role of physician experience and judgment.

Shared decision-making reflects and reveals the role of judgment and preference in practice variation,[32,33] and offers a role for patient preference to factor. Ideally, doctors recognize the importance of patients' opinions, explain the options, and invite joint discussion of those options to jointly arrive at a treatment decision.[34]

Though there is some debate about the impact of shared decision-making, such processes can lower health care costs and raise patient satisfaction. Studies show fewer hospitalizations and surgeries result when patients get enhanced support for making medical decisions,[35] and substantial cost savings from avoided surgeries.[36] Supported in shared decision-making, consumers often choose less invasive options,[37] suggesting potential cost savings if applied more often.[38]

One group is so committed to shared decision-making, they started a movement to foster it. The Society for Participatory Medicine's (SPM) founders—a diverse group of health care stakeholders—informally gathered for years to discuss how to make health care better, particularly in the face of rapid technological developments. They wanted to turn their discussions into reality and founded SPM.

Danny Sands, MD, SPM cofounder and current board chair, and assistant clinical professor of medicine at Harvard Medical School, defined the participatory medicine movement as one in which "patients and health care professionals actively collaborate and encourage one another as full partners in health."

A leading voice in this movement, SPM convenes patients, caregivers, and professionals to foster active collaboration.* "Open communication,

---

* In 2019, I joined SPM to support its mission.

sharing information, sharing in decision making. It's a mutual respect and trust, and then, finally, there's engagement," Sands explained. "Those are the elements of a successful collaboration in any realm." He hopes to see more application of these principles in health care. Too often, though, patient and provider interactions are like a car wash, in which the patient is the car and "they're passively cruising through that health care system carwash and getting health sprinkled on them and magically coming out the other end healthy." Sands would rather see true mutual engagement become the norm.

THE DIFFICULT PATIENT

When doctors do not invite shared decision-making, patients can feel they must push to participate in their care decisions. Some consumers I spoke to worried that, in their efforts to engage and be heard, they would be considered difficult patients. For months, "I was trying to tiptoe around other people's feelings and the fact that I was a medical student and didn't want to be this difficult patient," Priya told me. "[That] ended up delaying the care that I think I should have gotten for no reason."

Priya's arms had started tingling a day after helping her father build some furniture. Around that time, she was also waking up at night with her arms numb. Despite wearing braces for her hands and elbows thinking she had carpal tunnel syndrome, her symptoms got worse. Typing felt uncomfortable; she struggled to lift a book. When she noticed that she could feel the bathwater temperature with her toes but not her fingers, she realized she had a nerve issue. Tests ruled out autoimmune disorders and problems with her sensory and motor systems.

Consulting an orthopedic surgeon, Priya felt frustrated by his cursory exam and tennis-elbow diagnosis. "He pretty much just looked at me for a second and didn't do a neuro exam."

Though she didn't trust the surgeon's judgment, Priya followed his recommendation for physical therapy. After 10 weeks of physical therapy, she still struggled to chop vegetables or hold a phone to her ear. Now, she felt urgency. "I don't want to be difficult again, but something needs to be done because I can tell something is wrong."

When the orthopedic surgeon offered to refer Priya to a vascular surgeon, she felt he was pushing her along, out his office, and failing to look out for her. "I could see signs. I'm going to get ping-ponged around in this system for a couple more months until we figure it out."

Priya took a stand, surprising herself with how firm and direct she was. "I don't think this is a vascular problem," she said to the surgeon. "I think this is a nerve problem. I think we need to do a nerve test." The doctor agreed. "You're right," he acknowledged.

Looking back, Priya is glad she stood up when she did. "If I had gone with my 'I'm not going to be a difficult patient and I'm just going to listen to what they tell me,' I would have gone down a rabbit hole and not come to the conclusion that we did."

Why did this well-educated, well-informed patient care so much about not being seen as difficult? Priya felt she should defer to the surgeon's expertise and specialization. She also understood how frustrating it can be when patients come in armed with Google searches and demands for specific tests or treatments. "Being a medical student, I have seen patients when they come in and they're kind of demanding, and they have a certain attitude about what should be done." Physicians get turned off or annoyed by that attitude. "I just didn't want to be that to these doctors."

Suzanne Koven recognized the challenge for consumers in speaking up. "Patients are sometimes afraid to speak out because they don't want to be considered difficult, because then they think that they'll receive worse treatment," she said. "And they may be right about that."

Priya also validated these fears. "If you lose your credibility or someone doesn't want to listen to you anymore, once you kind of break that relationship, it's really hard to get them to get that person back on board." Because most patients are so reliant on providers to prescribe the right test or treatment, "you want them to believe you're credible and you don't want to be an annoying patient because you want them to do the right thing for you. You just want them to look out for you."

During Priya's neurology rotation in medical school, a patient had arrived with a pillow, complaining of multiple sclerosis symptoms. The pillow triggered assumptions on the clinical team that this patient was faking her symptoms. Doctors are trained to spot hypochondriacal patients by a "teddy bear test," in which adults present at the hospital seemingly overeager for an experience most people want to avoid and ready to settle in with the comforts of home. Though Priya and her colleagues were skeptical, they ran the necessary tests, which came back positive. If they had been negative, Priya is sure the clinicians never would have believed her again.

But some patients do exaggerate symptoms, and Priya had also seen that during her psychiatry rotation, once falling for a patient's manic act. "I understand why there is mistrust between docs and patients sometimes." As a future clinician, she hopes to develop judgment on whom to trust and how to give patients appropriate attention. "I personally hope to err on the side of caution and try to listen to people and hear them out."

STUPID BODY SYNDROME

For years, Paulette went to doctors for relief from pain whose source was hard to identify. "I had no idea what was wrong with me and they had no idea what was wrong with me." She coined her own mock diagnosis to explain how she felt. "I would tell physicians, 'I have Stupid Body Syndrome,' and they would laugh and say, 'That's a great name.' But they never had an answer for me."

Paulette never felt heard in these encounters. "They basically would ignore the questions I had because they couldn't answer them. It was very clear to me that if a physician did not know what was wrong with me and couldn't fix me, they didn't want to see me anymore. Because their job is to fix people and they couldn't fix me, it was very clear from their reactions, they did not want to see me." She was told by one doctor of her chronic pain, "I guess it's your cross to bear."

Following a tip from her physical therapist, Paulette saw a geneticist, who finally confirmed she has an often-missed genetic connective tissue disorder called Ehlers-Danlos syndrome. "I started crying because it was a huge relief. 'Oh my God, it's not in my head. It's something that's real.'" Now in her 60s, Paulette had suffered the effects of this disorder for at least 40 years. "I was taking 12 Advil a day for a long time, which obviously did a lot of damage to my insides, but that was because I could not get a doctor to recognize what was going on and take me seriously." Paulette paid physical—and psychic—costs from being undiagnosed.

Having a clear diagnosis increased Paulette's confidence. "I've seen so many bad physicians over the years, I just can't put up with them anymore. Understanding my diagnosis now gives me more backbone. It just makes me feel freer to question physicians, to not go back to them if they do not understand." She finds herself educating her other doctors about her condition and feels empowered to do so.

Being heard gave Paulette her voice. She uses her voice to get the right care for herself.

BEING HEARD

"There is no greater gift a doctor can give than saying, 'Tell me the whole story the way you want to tell it, and begin at the beginning, whatever that beginning is,'" Suzanne Koven said.

But doctors don't always give patients this gift. Time is their most obvious constraint. One study calculated the median primary care visit length to be 15.7 minutes.[39] Not only do doctors have "productivity" expectations—a number of patients they need to see in a day or an hour—but there are more administrative requirements on doctors as well. More than half of physicians report spending 10 or more hours a week on administrative tasks, and nearly 30% identify dealing with rules and regulations as the most challenging aspect of their job.[40]

"Compared to 15 years ago, there's simply more stuff I'll have to do that isn't taking care of patients," Koven said. Ironically, electronic medical records designed to improve efficiency have pushed a lot of clerical work onto doctors. "There is a drive to standardization and accountability that may have started out with good intentions," she continued. These rigid requirements aim to improve quality of care and to ensure consistency across patients, but many of those tasks fall to clinicians. And they take time.

Despite work-arounds and time-savers—like in-office scribes to take notes for doctors or telehealth visits to save time for doctors and patients— Koven says these approaches are "not addressing the fundamental fact, which is that taking care of people in the most traumatic, intimate, and complex experience of their lives takes more than 15 minutes."

Given those challenges, it's no wonder it can be hard to feel heard at the doctor's office. To avoid the kind of heartache and frustration—not to mention pain and expense—that Amanda, Paulette, and Ingrid experienced, consumer mind-sets and behaviors can increase the chance their health care voices are heard.

1. Don't worry alone

Doctors have historically been trained that over-diagnosing is better than missing a diagnosis. "If you're not taking out a few healthy appendices, you're missing some appendicitis," surgeons sometimes say.

The consumer equivalent of this philosophy is that it's better to ask too many questions than too few. If you're not sure you understand what the doctor is recommending, ask for clarification. If the doctor's plan doesn't feel right, ask if there are alternatives or what would happen if you didn't follow the recommendation.

For Rosemary, successful self-advocacy required great effort on her part. She had hurt her foot three years before our conversation. It wasn't healing quickly, so she went to the doctor for a follow-up visit on December 28 because the family had met their deductible for the year. "Take all the X-rays you're going to want," she had said. When she returned for follow-up care in January, they wanted her to do another series of X-rays. "It was six days later. And I refused. Let him look at the films they took six days ago," she suggested. Though the staff was adamant that the specialist wouldn't see her without new scans, the doctor wound up agreeing with Rosemary. New scans would have cost her hundreds of dollars unnecessarily. Rosemary had felt like crying but she stood her ground.

Speaking up does not always work. Tara questioned why she was having blood drawn at her first visit with a new PCP; though the doctor agreed it was unnecessary and promised to delete the order, the lab ran the tests anyway. "I was annoyed that I felt I had advocated for myself not to need something . . . and then even trying to eliminate what I thought were unnecessary tests . . . they were processed anyway."

Whatever the outcome, having raised concerns in the moment can give you more leverage in a dispute later than if you hold in your thoughts and concerns. Speaking up at least increases the chances you will be heard.

2. Ask for what you need

Suzanne Koven described seeing a doctor who did not look at her while he captured her information in the electronic medical record. "What you're doing right now doesn't feel good to me," she told him. He assured her once he input her data that the real visit would begin and he would turn his full attention to her. "But it'll be too late because I'm already anxious and mistrustful," she told him.

As hard as that was for Koven to say to a peer, she recognized how much harder it would be for most consumers. Yet, as a doctor, she told me how helpful it is to her when patients can express what they need. "I've had patients say to me, 'Look, this is really hard for me. What would really help me would be X.'" It's not necessarily a patient's responsibility, but it's helpful for doctors to know what's bothering you and what might help. "That's really helpful information to me," she said. Doctors want to feel effective and may appreciate your showing them how they might do so.

3. Get over your fear of being difficult

What's the worst that happens if you raise concerns or ask too many questions? You might feel silly or uncomfortable. Most Americans have been raised with a doctor-knows-best-inspired respect for physicians. We don't want to insult our doctors, make them angry, or cause them not to like us.

But Danny Sands emphasizes mutual respect. "The doctor may be an expert in their field of medicine. They have a lot of experience, a lot of wisdom to offer. But the patient is an expert in themselves and what they're going through and that should be appreciated. So, the doctor should respect the patient and the patient should respect the doctor."

Jerry, a former corporate executive who came out of retirement to serve in local government, had cared for his aging mother toward the end of her life: "It felt like asking questions implied confrontation, like second guessing versus getting information." He had the capacity to advocate for his mother and to ask questions respectfully. Still, he felt social pressure not to do so in the health care context. Despite that pressure, he did ask questions when he needed to.

Being the squeaky wheel can be uncomfortable, as people fear their questions reflect lack of respect for, or even mistrust of, doctors. What should consumers do to be heard and trusted rather than seen as difficult?

Is it worse to be viewed as difficult or to go without tests or treatment you might need? Ask yourself what the worst outcome could be of either scenario. The risk of annoying a doctor seems much lower stakes than the risk of missing a diagnosis. When it comes to your health, the stakes are just too high to worry much about being judged.

Consider a thought experiment in which the person who needs advocacy is not you but your child or parent, your grandmother, or best friend. I heard countless consumer stories about people's willingness to fiercely advocate for a loved one even when they reported passively accepting suboptimal care or treatment for themselves. Next time you need something, pretend you are advocating for your best friend. It may help you worry less about how you're perceived and focus more on making sure the right thing happens.

Priya suggested trying the physician's recommendations first but then speaking up if nothing improved or if there was no intervention at all. "It's very important for patients to advocate for themselves." But the first visit may not be the time to make demands or overly specific requests. Listen to your body, and if something is not right or you don't feel you're improving, it's time to speak up.

4. Recognize the art in medicine

Acknowledging gray areas in medicine might help consumers feel more comfortable asking questions and advocating for themselves. A single, established truth—or right answer—does not always exist. Jerry recognized this reality and would seek other sources for answers if he couldn't get what he needed from the doctors. "I did research on the side to figure out how much was art versus science." In the process, Jerry learned that a lot of medicine is actually art, which meant there were options, versus science, which meant "it is what it is." In the artful part of medicine, the consumer's preferences matter more. There are times when doctors—highly qualified, knowledgeable, good doctors—don't know the answer. Or there isn't an answer. There may be several comparable answers, not just one certainly right path. In those cases, using your voice is all the more important.

As discussed in Chapter 9, doctors do make mistakes. That's scary but also liberating in a way. It means you should trust your instinct and question doctors if you feel unsure that they're doing the right thing. Trust in doctors is often born of a belief that they have magical powers or at least that they know best. It can be soothing to believe that, especially when we're sick and vulnerable.

"Patients need to understand what their doctors are going through and that they're only human," Danny Sands advised, recognizing the high levels of physician stress, burnout, and even suicide.

Acknowledging doctors' time pressures is one way to show empathy. If you're scheduled for 15 minutes but your visit takes 45, that can throw off your doctor's day. Sands suggests balancing your own need to be heard by saying, "You know, doctor, I have something else I want to talk [about] with you, but I understand we're already over time. Should I make another appointment?" Avoid being demanding in that moment, he said. "It's not nice in any human interaction. [The] doctor's not your slave. And that's not going to work as well."

5. Do your part

Danny Sands contrasted the philosophy that "the customer is always right"—reportedly coined by the founder of Selfridges department store in the early 1900s—from Sy Syms, who famously used the slogan, "An educated consumer is our best customer."

Sands prefers the Syms approach. "Patients should take it upon themselves to learn about their illness. . . . They should actually demand [and] really expect that they can have access to the information they need so that [they] can understand their illness much better."

Going to the doctor and saying, "'I'm sick, doctor. Fix me,' That's not a good approach, medically, and it's just not going to work or get the kind of outcomes we want. A better approach is, 'Doctor, I'd love to partner with you so I can get myself better.'"

Sands encourages patients and doctors to plan ahead and set an agenda for each visit. Just as many doctors make plans for what to cover with patients, patients should do the same. "Prioritize that list because we've got to use this time effectively."

Participatory medicine, in which consumers are full partners in their health, need not take more time for doctors. It's better to have more time, but for it to work requires clinician openness to patient perspectives. Rather than telling patients to stay off the Internet, Sands suggests that doctors welcome patients who want to learn more and to not shy away from scheduling more time for discussion. "We can have a separate conversation about that. We don't have to fit that into the 15 minutes that we have scheduled today." As a consumer, ask for that time if you need it.

6. Seek diversity in your clinical team

Evidence suggests physician gender may matter more than the patient's for some clinical outcomes.[41] Women were more likely to die of heart attacks when treated by male physicians[42] and less likely to die or be readmitted to the hospital within 30 days of a hospitalization when cared for by female doctors.[43] In one study, just the presence of female physicians on the clinical team improved outcomes, even if they weren't the treating physician.[44]

7. Switch doctors who don't listen

If a doctor doesn't like your questions or conveys that he or she is not concerned about your situation, switch doctors. Like any relationship that doesn't make you feel good, it may be best to move on. Paulette reported having "seen too many physicians not willing to look outside the box, to think differently, to not listen, to not believe me." As a result, she is much more ready to vote with her feet. At a visit with her primary care physician, Paulette described how her doctor "never even looked at me. She sat at her computer asking me questions and writing down the answers. I thought, 'This is somebody who's clearly not interested in me,' and that was the last time I saw her."

We should assume that doctors are well trained and well intentioned. They want to provide the best possible care and to thoroughly address patient concerns and questions. But given the demands and time constraints of practicing modern medicine, consumers may need to be the squeaky wheel to make sure they get the best care. Imagine the worst outcomes if doctors don't devote the attention or energy to your concerns. Amanda could have died of a ruptured appendix. Paulette and Ingrid would have continued suffering for years longer. Rosemary would have gotten a sizable bill for repetitive scans; she might be able to absorb the cost but such expense would create true hardship for many people. These risks dwarf the risk of annoying the doctor whose schedule is packed with waiting patients, especially if you can trust that the doctor most likely wants to give you the time and attention you need to share your story as you want to tell it.

9

Don't You Know Who I Am?

How to define health care quality for yourself

"I have a really good dentist," J.J., a minister from New York, told me.

"How do you know?" I have, in the past, asked questions like this to challenge assumptions. But here, I was genuinely interested in how J.J. determined the quality of her dentist. How to measure real health care quality often confounds health care providers and insurers. Maybe J.J. had a better answer.

J.J.'s first response was what you might expect. "I've never had any problems with anything he's ever done." That seems like a good indicator of dental quality to me; I once ended up with a giant bruise on my face after a dental procedure.

But J.J. also took cues from what she called the "gestalt"—the general character—in the clinic. "The vibe is good. His relationship with his staff is good. The people who work there seem happy and appreciated." I've never seen employee satisfaction on any health care quality scorecard or rating system. But maybe it should have a place in health care quality measurement, especially if you subscribe to the iconic mogul Richard Branson's philosophy: "If you take care of your employees, they will take care of the clients."[1]

J.J. noted her dentist's manner. "He's straightforward. When he says he's going to do something, he does it." He narrates as he works, describing what he's doing as he does it. "People who are transparent are usually good," she said. Her dentist's openness instilled confidence and signaled competence.

In a nutshell, J.J. judged her dentist on three metrics: outcomes (i.e., "a lack of problems"), customer experience (based on a positive atmosphere), and transparency.

ELUSIVE OUTCOMES

Official health care quality definitions tend to emphasize health care outcomes or the results of health care services. The Institute of Medicine defines health care quality as "the degree to which health care services for individuals and populations increase the likelihood of desired health outcomes and are consistent with current professional knowledge."[2]

Outcome measures can also be unfair to doctors and beyond their control. Too many variables affect how patients do in their care. How sick was the patient to begin with? Did the patient follow the recommended treatment plan? How effective are those treatments anyway?

Because of these complexities, many doctors object to being judged on outcomes using simplistic methods. Often, doctors think their patients are more complex than average, like a Lake Wobegon effect where everyone is above average, and don't want to be measured alongside doctors with easier cases. Doctors who treat more acute cases may look like they have worse outcomes than peers with more straightforward patients, even if they are better clinicians and able to handle greater complexity. They are at least willing to treat tough cases, whereas some doctors or surgeons may avoid more complex cases for fear of depressing publicly reported quality scores.

Reporting that thoroughly accounts for these nuances might be too complex to present in a clear and straightforward manner that would be useful for the average consumer. The result is often a surface-level view of how good a doctor is, aimed more at high marks from regulators and credentialing agencies than at providing real insight to consumers facing a choice of health care providers.

Some consumers focus on outcomes when judging providers, though not as many you might expect. Because the outcome of his knee surgery was good, Ralph forgave a known weakness with the surgeon—his bedside manner. "His personality is such that he looks at you like he's fixing your car. There's no warm, cuddly. That didn't matter to me that much, because his skill as a surgeon was more important than his pampering me." The good result compensated for the lack of warmth.

But in a national survey about how Americans evaluate health care provider quality, only 11% cited the doctor's ability to accurately diagnose and fix their health problems.[3] Perhaps this number is so low because people simply assume their doctors can accurately diagnose and treat them.

A PREFERENCE FOR PROCESS

Instead of outcomes, health care organizations often measure procedural steps—Did the doctor ask the right questions? Inform the patient of certain options? Check the right boxes? These questions are easier to answer and quantify than whether the patients got what they needed.

Health plans spend lots of money and time meeting bureaucratic proxies for health care quality. The National Committee for Quality Assurance—the leading health plan accrediting body—measures health plan quality based on more than 90 standard measures,[4] including many process measures. For example, to combat obesity, health plans report on how often participating doctors assess patients' body mass index (BMI),[5] an important step in understanding whether doctors are paying attention to BMI, but not a measure of BMI itself, nor of whether obesity rates are improving or worsening.

Along the same lines, one of my health plan colleagues from the quality department once asked the marketing team to write a letter encouraging health plan members to stop smoking. Quality had promised our state regulator that at some point in the preceding 18 months, the plan would promote tobacco cessation. Time was almost up.

"We can write you a letter," I said, "but it's not likely to cause anyone to stop smoking."

"That's ok," my colleague replied. "We just have to do something because we said we would."

Wasn't the point to help people stop smoking? Why bother checking boxes with no hope of meaningful impact? But encouraging people to stop is an activity we could control; actually causing people to stop was much harder to achieve. And I was complicit, helping check boxes even as I knew the effort would likely have no material impact.

This experience illustrates Goodhart's law,[6] named for economist Charles Goodhart, which states that once a measure become a target for intervention, it ceases to be a good measure. People try to optimize performance on that measure, sometimes to the exclusion of other important aspects of performance. In short, people start gaming the system and lose sight of the real goal. In health care, it can be surprisingly easy to lose sight that the real goal is improving health.

In defense of real health goals, *Consumer Reports* began publishing hospital quality rankings. Years ago, I asked one of their health experts about physician objections to such rankings: How had they adjusted the scores for complexity and acuity? The expert explained they had based the rankings on patient safety and questioned how they might have appropriately discounted results based on patient complexity. Shouldn't hospitals maintain the highest safety standards, especially in the most acute situations? Still, the loudest complaints I heard about *Consumer Reports'* health care rankings were in private, from people at some of the institutions being evaluated.

Connie, a marketing consultant, tried to educate health care clients how to bridge the divide between their own definitions and consumer expectations of quality. "What does the consumer want out of you?" she'd say. "They want to *live*, for God's sake." Doctors and other professionals would argue, "But we're the best quality," to which Connie would respond: "If you have to say quality, then you're not quality. You'd better *be* quality."

When J.J. offered a clear—and very different—way of assessing her dentist than I had seen inside the industry, I wondered if consumers themselves might offer new ideas for measuring quality, based on what they care most about. So I asked. Here's what they told me.

IT'S HARD TO TRUST REVIEWS

Judging quality is not easy for consumers, just as it challenges health professionals. Fewer than half Americans surveyed felt it was easy to find health care quality information they could trust, and a majority said they rely on information from their friends or family.[7]

Despite the availability of online reviews to help consumers judge quality, those ratings can be unreliable and misleading. Sophie laughed when she admitted to using published rankings to choose new doctors after she and her husband moved across the country. When I asked why she laughed, she explained, "It's hard to tell how reliable they are. I think a lot of it is marketing. If you're a doctor and you really want to get on that list, there's probably some way to game the system."

"It's very hard to judge," Louisa told me. After a difficult labor with the birth of her daughter, she went to a chiropractor who "took a zillion different X-rays and made up a bunch of stuff and it didn't help at all." Her doctor later gave the chiropractor low marks for doing unnecessary scans and offering bad information, explaining that Louisa had bruising which would heal on its own. "It's hard to tell with outcomes, what's worked. Sometimes you can tell they're knowledgeable when you do your own research. Nowadays, you look online and see reviews and what others have said, and you look to your friends and see what they say." The chiropractor had not done anything of value for her, "but the guy had fabulous reviews."

Consumer satisfaction *is* important. As a patient, it is helpful to know that people like a doctor, that they feel heard, or that they can access or communicate easily with the doctor when they need to. But it may not tell the full story. For example, sometimes high-quality care is good care precisely because it doesn't give the patient what he or she wants. Lillian, a part-time nurse, addressed that not all dissatisfaction is based on reasonable expectations. "If I have a patient that all they want is that opioid prescription, they're going to be really not satisfied when I don't give it to them." Patients who want specific drugs they've seen advertised on TV don't always leave happy. "When you're trying to be customer-centered, it doesn't always work with the patient because what they're wanting is not sometimes appropriate and safe for them to have."

When I research restaurants or hotels, I look at the bad reviews. If a hotel isn't clean, I move on. But if reviewers are angry about the cost of valet parking and I won't be driving, I may book it. With any online reviews where measures are subjective, it is hard to know whether you share values and standards with other reviewers and, therefore, whether to trust their assessment. In health care, there can be so many factors, other consumers' reviews may simply not apply to your situation, characteristics, or preferences. That may explain why few Americans report putting a lot of stock into other consumers' ratings when choosing doctors.[8]

PROXIES FOR QUALITY

Because it is so difficult to measure health care outcomes or to judge quality overall, consumers use proxy measures to gauge health care quality.

Visual cues made an impression on Amanda, a young professional who had an emergency appendectomy detailed in Chapter 8. "This is what health care should be," she said of her inpatient experience. Almost sheepishly, she admitted the influence of being in a nice facility. "There were really superfluous luxuries of the stay. I'd be lying if I said they didn't play any role in my perception of quality."

Curtis, a businessperson from San Francisco profiled in Chapter 7, also judged the quality of his son's acute and rehabilitation care based, in part, on the overall consumer experience. He inferred quality from renovations that have made hospitals look like hotels or corporate lobbies—clean, new, and professional. Similarly, the supportive, empathetic staff conveyed good-quality care, especially when it is so hard to judge objectively. "That goes a long way to impacting one's opinion of the quality of what gets delivered. It's tough to say, would the outcome have been better or worse had he gone to the place down the street instead? I don't know."

When Hannah, a young woman who needed orthopedic surgery, chose a surgeon, she felt a doctor's credentials didn't tell the whole quality story. She valued "patient care," which she defined as "how they are as a person, how they interact with their patients. You could have the most impressive resume but if they ignore you and don't listen to your needs or concerns, that's not really the kind of doctor that I want to have." In a national survey,[9] more than half of consumers reported prioritizing interpersonal characteristics—like doctors who listen, are attentive, show interest, or have a caring attitude—when evaluating health care provider quality.

Even the perception of skill gave consumers confidence. Sean equated professionalism with competence. "I obviously don't have the content area knowledge to know just how high quality it was. But certainly, it felt professional, so it was positive."

When Emily struggled with infertility, she evaluated three specialists who had been recommended to her. She researched each one's credentials and patient ratings. The specialist she chose had high marks all around. He was the head of the practice and had an academic appointment, which she felt signaled up-to-date techniques. Also, "his patients said he was sympathetic and patient with them, and that felt like that's what you need at this point." Breaking into tears when she spoke of this doctor's empathy, Emily demonstrated just how important it was that he had "the perfect combination of both academic [credentials] and bedside manner."

Rapport invites open communication, which can lead to better care, as discussed in Chapter 8. Louisa reflected on her bad chiropractor's good reviews. "Some people judge by how nice they are, and do they listen," she said. Indeed, in the national consumer survey on judging quality,[10] two-thirds of consumers said ratings of a provider communications were important in their selection.

For Terri, the mother of three adult daughters, her doctor's personality put her at ease. "I want a doctor that is personable, that they can have a two-minute conversation about your life and remember things, even if he takes notes and puts it in his chart, and reads it. It does help to build rapport and make it comfortable so that you can feel like you can ask questions." When doctors or dentists are "all business," Terri felt "intimidated to even say anything."

Open communication was explicitly part of Adam's definition of quality. His daughters' pediatrician shares her cell phone number for after-hour and between-visit text messages. "The fact that we have that kind of access and you're not calling an answering service and then having the person get the message, and they'll call you back, that feels like a high level of care." The time the doctor spends with them gives him the same feeling. "That we can go in there and talk to her for an hour always feels almost luxurious." The office setup has a circle of chairs to enable conversation.

"That kind of experience really sets it aside from a much more procedural, clinical environment where it's like, 'come sit in this seat, put on a gown, we'll see you for ten minutes, now you're done.'"

FIT CAN DEFINE QUALITY

Certain services lend themselves to using interpersonal skills as a proxy for quality, where the fit between patient and provider may be more important than anything more tangible. In psychotherapy, for example, fit may be the best way to measure quality. "It's a little bit like a blind date," explained Hope, both a therapist and a patient. She might have two friends she likes a lot, but she can't be sure they'll like each other. "I can't speak to how the fit is going to feel, and you really need to pay attention to that," she advised. "Fit can look different for different clients, and clients need different things from us." Unlike surgery, where Ralph could overlook his skilled surgeon's terrible bedside manner, "for therapy, the bedside manner really matters more," Hope explained. Studies suggest fit, or "therapeutic alignment," matters most in how effective patients feel therapy is.[11]

For Adam, fit was also an important measure of quality. "The [pediatrician's] care is consistent with our values, and how we take care of ourselves and the role that medicine and drugs play even in our adult lives. The fact that there's consistency there and that we're not at odds with her says to us that this is high quality." Adam and his wife eat healthfully, avoid processed and high-sugar foods, and exercise. They vaccinate their children but are slow to medicate, often trying natural remedies before prescription drugs. It was important to them that their pediatrician be open to alternative approaches when appropriate. The doctor's emphasis on child development, nutrition, exercise, fresh air, and play fits their active and natural lifestyle. Their sense that she loves their children makes them love her.

Not only is this pediatrician's approach aligned with their personal values, but she reflects their social community as well. "There's a lot of people around us making the same decision. That says something in terms of the value and quality of health care they're receiving, too."

Where fit is unique to each patient–clinician match, that partnership can be an important marker of quality. "The good doctors sort of enlist you to help them with your treatment, as well as with your diagnosis," Jason reflected. His doctor partnered with him to manage the cost of his asthma medicine, recognizing cost as a top concern. "He understood that I didn't have a lot of money." The doctor gave Jason scenarios—what to do if this or that happened—so Jason would know what he needed to come in for and what he could safely manage on his own. Doctors agree with Jason; in a national physician survey, 75% said they prefer to share decisions with patents.[12]

FIT IS IN THE EYE OF THE BEHOLDER

Doctor–patient fit sometimes takes the opposite shape of classic consumer empowerment or shared decision-making. As described in Chapter 4, Ruby avoided making health care decisions. "My best doctors are the ones who don't make me figure it out," she explained. "It's not like a cafeteria where I have to know what I want and ask for the right thing. It's people who help me to spot what I couldn't spot myself and ask the questions to figure it out."

Leah, a cancer patient, similarly wanted her doctors to take charge. Though an avid researcher in other parts of her life, she did not look too closely into her diagnosis. "I have never Googled ovarian cancer," she admitted. "I just kind of let the doctors worry about that. I just feel like it's their job, they get paid the big bucks to think about this stuff and know about it, and then I just do what they tell me."

When a new doctor joined Leah's care team, he offered her new choices, which confused her. "I felt like it was patient-centered care to a point that it was becoming irritating. Don't make this my decision. I don't know anything about this and you all need to make this choice for me." Leah wondered why the new doctor's recommendations differed from her prior doctor's approach, and whose ideas were better. "I didn't understand why two doctors, with the same patient, in the same field—same everything—would have two different plans for me." She felt sure, "Somebody has a better idea. These ideas can't be equal." Unsure whom to trust or how to figure it out, she decided to trust the new doctor, finally asking, "What is the better choice? That's the choice I'm going to do. Can we just not make any more decisions here? Just tell me what to do and I'm going to do it."

Still other consumers may be put off by know-it-all doctors. "The thing that I love the most to hear in an appointment with a doctor is when they say, 'I don't know, let me check,'" said Sabrina, a researcher who also trained as an emergency medical technician.

Paulette also craved humility from her doctors. When we spoke, she was trying to get to the bottom of a digestive issue causing her to lose her appetite, even for chocolate, her favorite food. One gastroenterologist she saw "had no idea what to do." Another "tried lots of different things and he just couldn't figure it out." The second one admitted he didn't know what else to do, which Paulette loved to hear. "You can accept that you don't know. That, to me, is the mark of a great doctor." His willingness to admit defeat was endearing and validating, which was enough to satisfy her.

Louisa also appreciated when her gynecologist admitted she had failed to order a test Louisa needed. The doctor took responsibility and promised not to charge her to get the test done properly. This response increased Louisa's trust. "Sometimes you can see clearly when they make a mistake and when they don't take responsibility, it's not a good sign."

ASSUMING GOOD QUALITY

Many consumers simply expect that high-quality care is the norm. One study revealed consumers assume their doctors are meeting best-practice standards.[13] And organizations like state boards of registration in medicine and the Joint Commission on Accreditation of Healthcare Organizations exist to create and enforce quality care standards.

Ruby ascribed her lackadaisical attitude toward choosing a physician to this belief. "For standard care, I'm not worried about the quality of care. Maybe because I think of myself as a healthy person, I don't feel that I need someone who people say is the most knowledgeable. No, I just need somebody who's not unpleasant to be with."

"I don't buy into the notion that there are good doctors and bad doctors," Jerry told me. A former telecommunications executive, Jerry was influenced by his schizophrenic brother's experience. "I think it really matters most if they like you or not." Jerry had moved to Massachusetts after retiring and was surprised how much stock Bostonians seemed to put in quality rankings. "People stack rank things in Massachusetts more than I've ever seen. First best, second best, and so on." None of that resonated for Jerry. "They all have competent doctors and if I'm sick, I'll be taken care of." Optimistic, trusting, or simply respectful of the baseline quality all doctors are trained to provide, Jerry could not—or did not care to—seek fine distinctions between hospitals.

Like many consumers, Jerry trusted doctors because he assumed they all meet rigorous standards, and therefore, anyone practicing medicine must be basically competent. Most consumers make the same calculation, even if unconsciously, every time we step onto an airplane. Because all U.S. commercial airlines must follow strict quality standards enforced by the Federal Aviation Authority, there are not many meaningful differences in quality across carriers; those differences would be hard for the average consumer to identify. Consumers, therefore, must judge airlines based on measures they can directly experience. Quality of snacks, leg room and seat comfort, friendliness of staff, and reliability of the online applications therefore stand in for deeper quality measures.

Evaluating health care based on tangible measures is also reasonable, provided underlying quality meets high standards. How you feel in the doctor's office or about your hospital stay may be as important as tiny percentage differences in more technical quality standards.

Alexa explicitly chose doctors based on the assumption that her care would be good no matter who provided it. A young cancer survivor from Australia, she moved to the United States after going into remission. "I really prioritize finding doctors that are kind," she described her process to choose caregivers in her new home base. "Especially with cancer, it's very protocol-based. I think the treatment you're going to get between one provider and another is unlikely to change, so there's no real trade-off to find someone who's kind." When you trust that all doctors will follow the appropriate guidelines, why not choose someone nice?

GOOD CARE IS PERSONALIZED

Most health care experts view standardized, evidence-based medicine as the holy grail of health care quality. That is, highest-quality care derives from evidence of what has been proven to work in large clinical studies. Clinicians who follow these proven protocols are considered high-quality clinicians. Health care guru Atul Gawande promotes standardization in his *Checklist Manifesto*.[14] The less doctors improvise, the better.

Consumers, however, think of the best care as personalized: customized to their individual needs. Patients tend to assume that using evidence as the basis for treatment is the floor, not the ceiling. Research[15] shows that consumers assume it is rare for doctors to deliver substandard care, and they especially trust their own doctor's judgment. Consumers generally believe doctors are smart, good at their jobs, knowledgeable about evidence, and prone to follow it. Yet the best doctors go beyond the evidence, consumers believe, customizing their care to patient's individual needs. The very guidelines and standards experts believe ensure the highest quality of care seem to consumers to be overly rigid and likely to interfere with their physicians' autonomy and ability to customize care to them.

Customization is what consumers told me they wanted.

The physical therapist Ralph had seen after his first knee surgery "treats everybody the same" and not in a good way. Everyone went through the same protocol on the same schedule, without regard for their specific response. "I wanted somebody who was more attuned to the individual in terms of what help they needed." After his second surgery, Ralph chose a new physical therapist who based the treatment on Ralph's body. "I progressed at my rate of speed versus the generic rate of speed." It went faster the second time, and it was more pleasant. "I felt that the therapist was working on my body [with] a personalized approach." One size fits all had slowed Ralph's first recovery down; personalization led to a better outcome and greater satisfaction.

Andrea, a pancreatic cancer patient described in Chapter 7, was immensely frustrated with the limits of protocol-driven care. Her treatment was based solely on protocol. "As opposed to the surgeon taking into account your age, or your personal situation, the number of children you have, or other illnesses," Andrea was 37 years old with three kids under nine when she was diagnosed with the often-lethal cancer. The first-line chemotherapy did not shrink her primary tumor; the cancer actually spread. Potentially life-saving surgery was off the table at that point, and her prognosis was bleak.

"It's frustrating, because you feel like your situation is very personal to you, and it doesn't feel personal when you think that the doctors are making decisions based on data, as opposed to a person." Andrea found a nonstandard path to a promising drug, and it worked for her. Without challenging the standard of care for her cancer, she likely would have lost her battle.

Protocol-driven care does not always result in less or worse care. When 83-year-old Sam fell and hit his head, strict adherence to the protocol landed him in the hospital. "Every checkbox on the neurological check sheet was negative, except for my age. As a consequence, I got the fall diagnostic preventive treatment involving a CT-scan, overnight in the ICU, a lot of monitoring, all of which is according to protocol." He might not have needed all that attention, but the protocol called for an abundance of caution.

BLATANTLY BAD CARE

Sometimes, bad quality is blatant, and consumers can tell they are not getting personalized care. "It does not instill confidence," Sabrina said. When she called her primary care clinic for advice about her young daughter's hormonal abnormality, she felt it "was like a brick wall" and like they treated her daughter "as a piece of paper." Even as a health care insider, Sabrina struggled to decipher the best answer from the available evidence. "It was a question of needing to feel my daughter was being seen as an entire patient," she explained why she sought a second opinion from a top-rated academic medical center. "They did a complete physical exam. The doctor who I spoke with had actually read my daughter's chart."

In contrast, Sabrina had been to appointments for herself, her aging parents, or her children, where "it is immediately apparent that they have no idea who you are, or why you're there despite the fact that they have been given your information ahead of time and that they should have taken the care and time to read it." One nurse was confused why Sabrina's father was on a specific medication. Another time, Sabrina realized a doctor had given her mother a clean bill of health despite evidence to the contrary in her medical record.

Failure to read a patient's chart can lead to basic medical errors and reflects an egregious betrayal of one of the most basic aspects of listening, discussed in Chapter 8—knowing the patient and his or her specific situation. Sabrina understood why this failure happens. "They have ten minutes with you. They have 12 pounds of charting to do. They are running themselves ragged. It is not that they don't want to spend the time with you. They can't. But that doesn't mean they can't actually maybe look at your chart before they walk in."

In another case of egregiously bad quality, Terri's former dentist didn't demonstrate good hygiene. "That guy didn't wash his hands in front of me. And then he had his hands in his pocket. Then he worked, and I asked him about it. 'Why don't you wear gloves? Every dentist I've ever gone to wears gloves.'" He told her he couldn't work as well with gloves on, and Terri switched dentists as soon as she found a new one.

Likewise, Louisa's family doctor made clear errors. "I've reminded her my husband's allergic to penicillin and it's in his chart. But she prescribes it anyway. And when I correct her, she gets mad." The doctor had also given up on finding treatments for Louisa's difficult yeast infection. "I find it frustrating when a doctor gives you absolutely horrible advice and puts you on something that's proven ineffective," Louisa vented. "I could show you the studies that show it doesn't work for this. And you still go through the pain and you still have to pay the doctor. Other products you could say, 'This product doesn't work,' and get your money back. There should be some kind of accountability."

Art also received bad quality care and wished for someone to take accountability for the outcome. He had been struggling with longtime sinus problems when he finally felt his situation was urgent. "The entire right side of my face shut down," Art explained. "There was no air going through at all. It felt like I was suffocating." An emergency room doctor told him he needed surgery for strep and staph infections. "You are getting zero air through," the doctor told him.

Art wanted to get the surgery done at the closest academic medical center, which he assumed would be the best because they do the most procedures and have the best reputation. But he couldn't get an appointment, even to be evaluated, for three weeks. He went online and found a surgeon in his insurance network whose schedule was so flexible he answered his own phone and offered immediate appointment slots. Desperate for relief, and comforted by the surgeon's credentials, Art booked the surgery. "At this point, I don't really have a choice because I can't breathe."

The surgeon "sounded like he knew what he was talking about. If you don't know, all they have to do is throw around some medical terminology."

If one of Art's kids needed care, he said, "I research the shit out of it." But for himself, Art was convinced by the surgeon's apparent familiarity with the procedure and by his hospital-admitting privileges, which Art interpreted as an implied endorsement.

"I probably should have asked, 'How many times have you done this?' But I think he already told me he had done it 100 times. I had no way to validate whether that's true or not. They all say that they've done it a ton of times, that the surgery is easy. Nobody is going to say, 'It's the first time I've ever had to deal with this.'"

Three months after the surgery, the crisis had abated, but Art didn't feel much better and he would need another surgery to repair the initial work. "I think I had some red flags there. The guy simply had too much availability. It's Monday morning. I call the office at 8:30 to see if I can get in. The doctor himself calls me back and says, 'I have an opening at nine, 10, 11, and 12.' That's a red flag." He had wondered if he could get by with antibiotics and avoid surgery but found it hard to leave once he met the surgeon. "A lot of people, once they go see a doctor, they're hesitant to switch doctors. They feel bad. They just for some reason feel this affinity that if they go to get a second opinion, they feel guilty."

Adding insult to injury, Art still had $5,000 of outstanding bills from the surgery and would likely need to pay more for the revision surgery. "If I was not happy with another service," he said, "I wouldn't pay the bill. I would fight the bills. In this case, I have scar tissue that is causing me problems. I still can't breathe. Why am I still on the hook?"

THE QUALITY PYRAMID

Having heard many consumer definitions of quality—good and bad, I wanted to know how forward-thinking health care leaders defined it. Experts and insiders offered quality definitions focused on health care that is appropriate, accessible, timely, holistic, efficient, connected, equitable, and empathic.

One expert I consulted was Malaz Boustani, MD, MPH, a practicing physician, professor, and visionary at the Indiana University School of Medicine.* He spends his days working to transform what he calls "Health

---

* Malaz Boustani, MD, MPH, holds several appointments, including Richard M. Fairbanks Professor of Aging Research, Indiana University School of Medicine; Founding Director and Chief Innovation & Implementation Officer, Sandra Eskenazi Center for Brain Care Innovation; and Founding Director and Chief Innovation & Implementation Officer, Center for Health Innovation and Implementation Sciences at the Regenstrief Institute, and Indiana University School of Medicine

Care 1.0" into "Health Care 2.0." As the founding director and chief inno-vation and implementation officer at the Center for Health Innovation and Implementation Sciences, he trains and mentors the next generation of health care leaders, aiming to create an army of quality improvement change agents embedded in health care institutions.

"I'm so ashamed," Boustani told me, the anguish so deep in his voice I felt he was about to confess some personal transgression. The source of his shame was "the current quality of the service of Health Care 1.0."

Three pillars—safety, personalization, and precision—are critical to delivering the highest-quality health care, yet all currently represent improvement opportunities, according to Boustani. "Fundamentally, we make a lot of mistakes." He estimated that mistakes happen in one out of three, four, or generously, ten health care encounters. Personalization is lacking as well. "We treat the average, which doesn't exist in reality. It's a math concept that humans created, so there is not much personalization at all." Finally, he bemoaned the lack of evidence underpinning health care treatment today. "Our ability to tell you, 'This is the real signal,' we don't do that very well."

Safety is foundational, like the base or the floor—the minimum require-ment for health care quality—he explained. "In that safety, I want us to be at least as good as airlines, meaning, we can just make one mistake out of a million of our transactions." Our conversation took place soon after sev-eral fatal crashes caused the worldwide grounding of Boeing's 737-MAX. Health care errors happen with far greater frequency than aviation catas-trophes, yet because health care mistakes are so routine, we almost expect—and thereby tolerate—them. We should attend to improving health care safety with the same collective energy or urgency we apply to preventing more visible disasters.

On top of safety is personalization. "After we give you safe [care], the quality is defined by the consumer of our services." As a geriatrician, Boustani has patients who want to live forever and don't object to heroic measures to keep them alive; life itself is precious to them. "Ironically, I'm one of these people," he laughed. "I don't want to die, period. So I can sac-rifice pain and everything else. I'm willing to take that one per 10,000 chance that this could keep me alive, even if that means I go bankrupt."

But in his practice, he also sees patients on the other end of the spec-trum. For these consumers, "One day of pain free, one day of no hunger, one day of no thirst, one day of no anxiety, one day of no depression, and one day of meaning, it's worth years of suffering." They don't want Boustani to keep their heart beating at all costs. They say, "I just want to have that beautiful, meaningful interaction."

Rounding out the quality pyramid for Boustani is precision. "What is the evidence that that is actually the real signal, not a noise?" a reference to

Nate Silver's *The Signal and the Noise*,[16] about extracting real insights from vast amounts of data. Clinical recommendations should be filtered through the consumer's own values but based on evidence of the likelihood that they will deliver positive outcomes.

Boustani wants health care to emulate the best models for each of these three principles. For safety, "we have to learn from nuclear manufacturing and airlines." For personalization, "we have to be Ritz Carlton." For precision, "we have to be scientists. We have to be [National Institutes of Health]." Integrating these three ideas, Boustani wants to see precision that puts customers first. "It's all about customer value."

DOES QUALITY MATTER?

Like Ritz Carlton customers, consumers may be willing to pay more for higher-quality health care. Nearly two-thirds (64%) of Americans surveyed said they would be willing to pay more to see a higher-quality doctor. Costs matter, too, when choosing health care providers, but the edge goes to quality.[17]

"I may be cheap about certain things," Ralph admitted. A true negotiator as profiled in Chapter 6, he always seeks a better deal. "But other things, I am not cheap on. If I feel I have a quality doctor on something that I need to get fixed, then I'll pay a higher amount of money." Neither would he skimp on brakes and tires. "Most other things, I don't like paying, but I think those are two important things, and you need them. You need to be safe."

I met several consumers with enough means to prioritize quality over cost. "There isn't a price tag," Sabrina said of the second opinion she sought for her daughter. Her insurance company wouldn't cover the consultation with a top-rated hospital. It didn't matter to Sabrina. "If they had told me it's $20,000, I might have said, 'Maybe we don't need a second opinion,' but honestly, I probably would have put that on a credit card. I can't put a price tag on that."

Luckily, the bill was not $20,000, and Sabrina was able to pay it. "I don't make all that much money," she explained. "I work at a university and I'm supporting my two kids. We live paycheck to paycheck. I often feel like I should pay a little closer attention to what's coming in and what's going out than I do." But that's not her whole financial story. Sabrina's lack of focus on her finances is a mix of privilege and prioritization. She has savings that cushion her otherwise tight finances, and she prefers to focus on other things. "I'm of the opinion that my time is worth something."

Sabrina gave up on getting the visit covered. It didn't bear on her decision, so it wasn't worth her energy. "There was never a question in my mind that I wasn't going to get a second opinion because I have resources." In the end, that second opinion swayed her decision on which treatment path to pursue, an option she realized would not be available to many. "I kept thinking, 'What if I didn't have those resources?'"

Sabrina's philosophy applied to her own psychotherapy as well. "If I want to see my therapist, I'm going to go to my therapist. It doesn't really matter to me what that copay, or what the deductible is because I'm going to pay it either way. Whether my insurance covers 80% of it after $3,000 or 20% after $3,000, or doesn't cover it at all, probably isn't going to change my decision, if I believe it to be a good medical decision."

Simone similarly had the resources to buy the best health care possible. A filmmaker based in New York City, she had had a major health event more than a decade ago: a stroke in her 30s. She spent 10 days in the hospital and 18 months in follow-up care. She also has a family history of breast cancer, and the genetic predisposition to get it herself, so she was in a monitoring program. "I'm sure it contributes to this desire for really quality health insurance and willingness to pay for it."

The neurologist who treated Simone after her stroke urged her to get a primary care doctor who could help quarterback her care, given the complexity ahead for her health care life. That suggestion led Simone to a primary care doctor who is so good, "people kind of worship her." Whenever the primary care doctor refers her to other doctors, Simone feels she gets outstanding care because of that respect for her doctor. "It just feels worth it to me."

The doctor does not take any insurance, so Simone pays $300 per visit out of pocket. Simone has explored alternatives because of the cost, and the inconvenience of traveling 45 minutes or an hour across Manhattan to see her. But Simone won't switch. "I have tried a couple other doctors and networks and I just feel like she's worth it."

JUDGE FOR YOURSELF

How should *you* judge health care quality, given all the ways consumers think about health care quality—and how different some of those ways are from industry-standard measures, not to mention how hard it is for consumers to find trustworthy sources of quality information?

Health care quality is complicated—difficult for consumers to assess and for professionals to measure. Official industry methods for capturing and assessing health care quality are imperfect and challenging to implement.

Health care will get objectively better. Evidence will improve. Therapeutic options will expand. Data will illuminate real differences between better and worse options—treatments, providers, and facilities. Underlying improvements should also improve quality measurement and the presentation of quality results. Taken together, rules of evaluating health care quality should move beyond process-only measures and general rules of thumb like picking surgeons who do more procedures.

In the meantime, within the basic minimum quality thresholds and standards, the most important definition of quality is your own.

10

Should My Boss Control
My Health Care?

Untangling health insurance from employment

Lauren, an entrepreneur, credited her access to health insurance under the Affordable Care Act for her ability to take the risk of starting her own firm. "That was one of the factors that helped me make the decision to leave my job," she explained. Her husband was also self-employed, so neither had access to traditional employer-based insurance.

"The problem with health care is that if you wind up in the hospital, or you have cancer, it could be $100,000. It can ruin your life." If that were to happen, she assumed she or her husband would need to get a job with health benefits. "We'd have to give up our businesses to find a corporation that offered it. I feel like that's anti-American."

For Bianca, the wife of an entrepreneur, the ACA also represented financial opportunity. Being able to buy insurance directly, rather than needing to get it from an employer, "absolutely enables my husband to start this company. And I think how many people will he employ."

Her husband had previously launched a company in their living room that grew to employ 400 people across three cities. After he sold that business and wound down his obligations to the new owners, he officially started another new business. "He doesn't have a college degree. To make money, he has to do it himself," Bianca told me.

Bianca, herself, scarcely uses medical care. "I've probably gone to the doctor once in the last three years. . . . Even with insurance, I'm not the kind of person who runs to the doctor." Still, she was thrilled to have coverage, believing in the importance of having protection against downside risk. "I look at it as insurance—it's for something catastrophic." Also, she has children. "It's there as peace of mind, especially with kids."

UNLOCKING EMPLOYMENT

Comprehensive, quality health coverage was previously reserved for those with generous employee benefits and people old enough to qualify for Medicare or with income low enough to qualify for Medicaid.

The ACA—and Massachusetts health reform before that—made it possible for individuals to buy comprehensive yet reasonably affordable health insurance without being in one of those situations.

Under Massachusetts health reform, one of the first newly eligible members to sign up with the health plan I worked for was a 28-year-old woman. She had not seen a PCP in 10 years—her entire adult life. Like many consumers we met in those early days, this woman did not have the sort of employment situation that afforded her health coverage. In focus groups, we encountered a comic book store owner, a graduate student, a job seeker, and a seasonal worker, among others. None could have qualified for free Medicaid coverage, because their income wasn't low enough given their family structure. Medicaid is widely thought to be a benefit for anyone who is low income, but, in fact, it was designed for especially vulnerable populations, such as low-income children and their caregivers, and pregnant women. Before Medicaid expansion, single or childless adults could not necessarily qualify even with very low incomes.[1]

I wrote about these and other consumers' stories in TheHill.com[2] in 2017. I argued the business case for ACA health insurance marketplaces: access to affordable, high-quality health coverage enables entrepreneurship, which in turn fuels the U.S. economy. In 2018, more than 30 million small businesses employed nearly 60 million Americans, almost half the workforce.[3] Small businesses created nearly two million net-new jobs, with more than half coming from firms with fewer than 20 employees.[4] While Republican politicians had focused on repealing the ACA, I argued they might inadvertently squash entrepreneurship and small-business ownership.

Economists agree. As many as 15% to 20% of workers might shift to self-employment if access to health insurance were not tied to their employment, implying that two to four million more people might start businesses.[5] One study showed a small but statistically significant increase in self-employment among 65-year-olds, presumably emboldened by new access to Medicare.[6]

Stunted entrepreneurship is just one form of job lock. Economists also refer to labor-market distortions, in which people hold onto jobs they might otherwise leave for fear of losing access to comparable health benefits. Others may retire or choose to work part-time with access to health insurance.[7] For example, people with access to retiree health benefits were more likely to retire before age 65, resulting in 10% fewer working years for people with benefits compared to those with none.[8]

More generally, people with employer-sponsored health insurance stay at their jobs 16% longer and are 60% less likely to voluntarily leave their jobs than people with insurance through other sources.[9] As noted, employer-based insurance is estimated to reduce mobility by 15% to 20%, though individual studies find numbers ranging from no effect to a 50% reduction, depending on conditions and worker characteristics.[10]

Employees who feel locked into their jobs, clinging to specific employment-based coverage, may not pursue their passions, seek new challenges, or leave unconstructive work environments. Lauren and Bianca's husband would likely not have started their own companies, limiting their career satisfaction, financial opportunities, and contributions to U.S. economic growth—and, likely, their contributions at work. The productivity of unhappy employees suffers; happy employees are up to 20% more productive than unhappy employees.[11] Feeling locked in has detrimental effects on employees' well-being, including self-reported perceptions of health and even depressive symptoms.[12] Employers who use generous benefits to attract and retain the best candidates may inadvertently do too good a job at keeping people, some of whom should not stay.

Even with new options available via the ACA health insurance marketplaces, many employees remain stuck, locked into unsatisfying jobs because of fear they cannot fully replace their benefits.

Caitlin, a professional with a high-power corporate marketing job who had recently had her second baby, experienced this phenomenon. "Part of the reason I didn't leave my job before having a baby was like, 'This is an amazing health insurance, and I will have everything covered, and if anything goes wrong or anything, I don't have to worry about it at all.'" Caitlin was not alone in feeling she had to stay in a job for the benefits. "I literally had conversations with friends I work with that are like, 'We really want to quit our job, but if we want a second baby, does it make more sense to stay than to leave?'" Caitlin's calculus was explicit: "Do I stay longer in a job that I'm not crazy about because it offers such an incredible health care package? And I know that I'm very unlikely to get something this generous in terms of the health care coverage even if I have another good job that offers pretty good coverage."

A job has to be pretty miserable to leave such generous benefits behind, especially if you anticipate needing health care services in the relatively near future. Caitlin's employer is probably thrilled to keep her, but in a perfect world, its employees would be just as thrilled to stay. Generous health benefits are a gift, but one that locks both employees and employers into suboptimal employment arrangements.

HOW WE GOT HERE

People may assume employment-based health insurance is the bedrock of the U.S. health system, around which all other elements have been built. Yet, employment-based health insurance is a relatively recent phenomenon in American society.

Today, 56% of Americans get private health insurance through their employer,[13] a sizable proportion though a far cry from universal. Before World War II, however, only 12 million[14] people—or 9% of Americans—had health insurance at all, and private coverage was virtually the only type of insurance one could have.

Not as many people had, nor needed, health insurance because medical care was substantially less advanced in that era. Hospitals were often associated with death, rather than effective treatment, and medical care overall was more about comfort than cure.[15] The American College of Surgeons (ACS) was formed in 1913 to develop hospital standards and improve hospital quality through standardization. When the ACS surveyed 692 U.S. hospitals with 100 beds or more, not even 13% could meet the minimum standards ACS had set.[16]

Medicine advanced with improved standards and training. Physician influence and status rose, as did health care prices. In 1929, the average medical expense for an American family was $103, or about 5% of average annual income.[17] That year, Baylor University Hospital contracted with a group of Dallas school teachers to provide up to 21 days of hospital care in exchange for 50 cents per month from each participating teacher. Perhaps the first prepaid health plan, this arrangement smoothed out payment of potential future hospitalizations and provided the hospital with steady, predictable income in the Depression-era downturn. This concept spread; by 1937, there were 26 such plans covering 600,000 people.[18] More broadly, 1.2 million employees plus 1 to 2 million dependents were reportedly covered by employer-based plans by 1930.[19] Attracted by the financial benefits of insuring groups of younger, healthy, employed workers, insurers saw new business opportunities in the employer market.

If improvement in health care quality was one of the contributors to the growth of health insurance, World War II accelerated the process and tied it to employment. During the war, military service abroad created labor shortages at home. Fearing that unfettered inflation would result from rising wages in the tight labor market, Congress passed the Stabilization Act of 1942, and, based on powers resulting from that legislation, President Roosevelt issued an executive order freezing wages.[20]

Though complaining about the wage freeze was considered unpatriotic during the war, employers still worried about their ability to retain workers. Participation of women in the workforce jumped from 27% to 37% between 1940 and 1945 to fill gaps created by men serving in the military.[21] However, labor shortages persisted. Originally both a concession to workers feeling the pinch of these inflation-fighting wage restrictions and a business strategy to attract scarce labor, employment-based health insurance was born.

The Revenue Act of 1942 applied huge taxes to corporate profits to support war efforts, yet also allowed employee benefits to count as corporate expenses, offsetting profits. A 1943 IRS ruling that employees similarly did not need to pay taxes on employer-provided benefits further solidified the appeal of employment-based health insurance.[22] Following the war, with the U.S. economy booming, corporations continued offering health benefits to workers.

By 1950, nearly 77 million people—or 51% of Americans[23]—had health insurance. By 1959, 67% of Americans had hospital insurance, which rose to 81% by 1968.[24] And by 1970—following advances in medical treatment, dramatic increases in the number of hospitals and available beds, the advent of Medicare and Medicaid, and increasing medical costs—more than 175 million Americans, or 86% of the population, had health insurance.[25]

In other words, widespread health coverage, which we have come to think of as foundational to the American health care system, is a relatively modern development. Still, employer-sponsored health insurance has been around long enough for its limitations to reveal themselves. The modern-day employment-based system leaves people especially vulnerable—financially and clinically—when they lose a job, retire, or cannot work due to their own or a loved one's illness.

LOSING BENEFITS WHEN YOU NEED THEM MOST

By the time Kiri's employer informed him that it was dropping the family from its group health insurance plan, the employer had already done more than required by law. Kiri had been diagnosed with stomach cancer nearly a year before, rare in an otherwise healthy, fit man in his 30s. Kiri had undergone aggressive treatment, with initially promising results, and returned to work. But when his cancer stopped responding to available chemotherapies, he had a large part of his stomach removed and faced numerous complications with repeated emergency room visits and hospitalizations.

When the notice of benefit cancellation arrived, he was on the 8th floor of one of the country's most prestigious—and expensive—hospitals, for what would be his last admission.

Kiri was lucky, financially speaking. Living in Massachusetts—a politically blue state with a generous health insurance design—he and his family were able to qualify for subsidized coverage. Without his income, they could not afford to buy private coverage. Because of his cancer, they might not have been able to buy private insurance at all were it not for the protections of people with preexisting conditions.

This story highlights one of the greatest cruelties of American health care: when you're sick, can't work, and need health insurance the most, you're at greatest risk of losing coverage. Consumers at their most vulnerable should not have to depend on their employer's altruism to determine if they can keep health coverage when they need it most.

It also raises an important question: is it time to untangle health insurance from employment?

UNTANGLING HEALTH CARE AND EMPLOYMENT

The future of work is upon us.

The circumstances that gave rise to the modern employment-based health insurance system are no longer in place. Where there was little to spend health care dollars *on* a century ago, those limited health care treatment options and modest costs have been bulldozed by scientific advancement and medical inflation.

Labor shortages from an acute event—World War II—have given way to low unemployment, in part, resulting from worker skills gaps. In 2018, there were 7 million open jobs and just 6.3 million unemployed people looking for work. More than one-third of recruiters cited challenges finding candidates with the right skills or experience.[26] Better benefits might help firms draw skilled workers from other firms, but benefits alone will not create requisite talent pools where they don't exist.

The nature of work and relationships between employers and employees is completely different just two generations since the employment-based health insurance system developed. Long gone are the days of lifetime employment, pensions, and a true social compact between employee and employer built on loyalty and consistency. Corporations now seek greater agility and efficiency. Today's workers value mobility, flexibility, and variety.

According to a 2018 Gallup report,[27] one-quarter of U.S. full-time workers and half of part-timers have an alternative work arrangement as their primary source of income; 36% of U.S. workers participate in the gig economy in some capacity. Diane Mulcahy's *The Gig Economy*[28] suggests earning a living via nonstandard work arrangements can enhance financial flexibility and satisfaction, giving workers more control in living according to their individual values and priorities.

As more people participate in these types of work arrangements, the nature of work will continue to evolve. The Rand Corporation[29] summarizes a confluence of trends that they predict will influence the U.S. labor market in coming years. Slower workforce growth will continue to yield tight labor markets, in turn leading to greater labor-force participation among historically underrepresented demographic groups like women, older people, and people with disabilities. The pace of technological development will accelerate. Firms will increasingly specialize more narrowly and partner or outsource noncore functions. Employees will work in more decentralized arrangements. Weaker ties between employment and fringe benefits could result from enhanced productivity and associated rising wages.

As workers crave and demand more flexibility, benefits will also need to become more portable. The Society for Human Resource Management predicts the rise of more flexible, more personal health-related benefits.[30] For example, they suggest that more employers will offer health savings instruments like those defined in Chapter 11. The world in which employment-based health insurance was born is rapidly becoming a relic, and adaptation is afoot.

BREAKING THE CYCLE

Adaptation to new labor-market conditions is critical as the employment-based health insurance system strains under the weight of these changes. Americans may be starting to see the end of the seemingly inextricable link between employment and health insurance.

The value of employer-sponsored health insurance has been steadily eroding over the past decade, as discussed further in Chapter 13. That is, while employer costs have increased, employee costs have increased even more. Employers contribute a smaller proportion of insurance costs. Between 2009 and 2019, employee contributions to health benefit expenses rose approximately 70%, compared with a 50% increase in employers' share.[31] As a result, more of employees' income goes to paying premiums: the average employee premium contribution was almost 7% of U.S. median income in 2017, up from just over 5% in 2008.[32] Making matters worse, since 1999, health care premiums for people with employer-sponsored health insurance have risen more than three times faster than wages.[33] Economists estimate that every dollar employers spend on employee health benefits is approximately a dollar that doesn't make it into employee take-home pay. Workers may feel wage stagnation without realizing that a main cause is rising health costs.[34]

Along with higher premiums, 82% of employees now have deductibles, and deductibles are rising—estimates range from $1,700[35] to $1,800 on average nationwide.[36] Consumer satisfaction erodes as insurance value erodes. Those with the highest deductibles—$3,000 or more—rate their health plans the worst,[37] and half report health insurance has gotten worse in the last five years.[38]

Together, these costs create financial vulnerability for Americans with little or no savings. Estimates range from 29%[39] to 58%[40] of U.S. households having less than $1,000 in savings; another estimate suggests 40% of households have no savings at all.[41] One in six employees report having made "difficult sacrifices" to pay health care costs in the past year;[42] 40% had difficulty affording health care costs;[43] and half had postponed or fore-gone medical care or tests.[44] One in five people said health expenses had eaten up all or most of their savings.[45]

Angela, the mother of four with employer-based benefits, experienced financial strain firsthand because of her family's $8,000 deductible. "How in the world do you expect anyone to absorb this?" In Angela's world, employer-provided health insurance is better than nothing but nowhere near the protective benefit it once was.

LETTING GO OF EMPLOYER-BASED COVERAGE

For everything that is suboptimal about tying health insurance to employment, it would not be easy to unwind. First, any change to a system serving 158 million[46] people would cause upheaval and disruptive consequences. For all its flaws, the current system is at least well understood and enmeshed in the fabric of the American economy. As Aaron Carroll said in *The New York Times*, "Americans seem to prefer the devil they know to pretty much anything else."[47]

Such a shift is possible if employers revamped compensation, insurers expanded offerings, and consumers embraced taking charge of their health benefit selection.

Adjusting the current balance of wages and benefits would not be easy, though. Where would health coverage come from, and who would pay for it? Would replacing benefits with wages net a fair exchange? Would the increase in wages be sufficient for employees to buy their own health insurance? And are consumers ready and willing to take charge of their health benefit selection?

Converting benefits to wages, for example, would require employers to reconfigure compensation and benefits policies and staffing. Employers could provide funds that employees could use to buy insurance, using a "defined contribution" model in contrast to "defined benefit" plans. Defined contributions replace set benefits with a specific dollar amount, an allowance with which employees can buy their own coverage. This approach allows consumers to choose best-fit plans rather than forcing them into whatever plan their employer chooses to meet the employer's overall needs.

Jared, an individual health insurance buyer between jobs, was surprised that more employers have not embraced the opportunity to shift employees to defined contribution plans. "I would have thought that they would have given you dollars to go buy your health insurance on the exchange." The insurance marketplaces enable shifting "from employers making the decision and pushing it over to the individual." But, this approach would place the burden—and opportunity—of shopping for health insurance onto individuals.

With more individual shoppers for best-fit insurance plans, the market could theoretically create pressure on insurers to deliver better value and possibly lower-cost products.[48] Insurance options would need to exist, via accessible marketplaces. Insurers, not known historically for their embrace of innovation—or of the individual market, which tends to be less lucrative than selling insurance to large groups—would need to adjust offerings and respond to new market dynamics and customer demands. And individual insurance marketplaces, themselves, would need to thrive. However, the future of these health insurance purchasing platforms is subject to political forces; the resulting uncertainty puts insurance company participation at risk.

Another challenge with migrating to defined contribution plans involves demographics. Economists and advocates of defined contribution plans typically cite the young, healthy employee who might be able to pocket the difference between what an employer contributes to health costs and what the employee actually needs to spend. But what about older or less-well workers, who may have to pay more on their own to get sufficient coverage?

Tax rules that have long favored the current system of employer-provided health insurance would also need to change. The Revenue Act of 1918[49] specified that health insurance benefits—which very few Americans received—were not considered taxable income. In 1943, the IRS deemed health insurance provided by employers as not taxable to employees. After an IRS reversal in 1953, Congress reinstated the exemption. While the impact was initially negligible, now that employer-sponsored insurance is so prevalent, this tax rule amounts to a huge reduction in payroll and income taxes—approximately $250 billion per year of lost federal tax revenue.[50] The additional federal revenue from reinstating this tax could fund an expansion of the health safety net or allow a more targeted tax break.

Employees benefit from increasingly valuable health insurance as a form of untaxed compensation, though few may fully realize the trade-off it represents with wages. Employers can deduct health insurance costs as business expenses and sidestep payroll taxes that would otherwise apply if benefit costs were converted to cash compensation.

Some economists believe this tax shelter spurred demand for health benefits that stretched far beyond what catastrophic coverage for high-dollar, rare events health insurance was intended to cover. Expanded benefits that also paid for routine care in turn helped drive health care costs up and solidified the blocking effect of premium increases on suppressing wage growth.[51]

A PATH FORWARD

Even if we could, *should* we untangle employment and health care?

You probably wouldn't want your employer choosing where you go on vacation or how you decorate your home. Yet that's what's happening in employer-sponsored health insurance. The employer is shopping for health insurance but not directly on your behalf. The employer makes the best decision it can for the entire organization, balancing overall costs with what employees will tolerate. Employers must think about the total pool of employees and balance the needs represented within that pool. The highest-cost, highest-need employees may not fully get the coverage they need, while the lowest-utilizing employees may pay more than necessary to meet their own needs. Companies aim their health benefit selections at some common denominator of employee needs. By definition, therefore, employers do not and cannot optimize for each individual's needs.

It seems clear that the current system is suboptimal, with employers providing cookie-cutter plans—the most generous of which likely overspend relative to what many employees need, the less generous of which leave many people painfully exposed, financially. The current system is expensive and unsustainable and out of date for the modern workplace. Decoupling employment and health insurance would put more responsibility onto consumers, which not all consumers want. But it might be worth the effort to have more direct control over health insurance selection and a more direct way to signal the market about needs and preferences. If consumers demanded this decoupling—along with requisite tools and insurance options to make such a transition work—the result could be a healthier, more competitive market. And more consumers would likely get coverage that better suits them.

11

Speak Our Language

How jargon keeps consumers out of the loop, and
how to reclaim the language of health care

"What's a deductible?" Noah remembered asking himself on his first visit
to Healthcare.gov to find an individual insurance plan he could afford.
A graduate student, he had no access to a large employer-sponsored health
plan and he was too old to stay on his parents' plan. He had never bought
his own health insurance before.

Most Americans—158 million[1]—get their health insurance through
their employer, as discussed in Chapter 10. This large swath of the population has scarcely needed basic health insurance literacy. Their employers
curate health insurance choices—if they have any choices at all. Yet, as
health plan designs shift more financial responsibility onto individuals
and families, even those with employer-provided coverage need more
competency in navigating health insurance.

The need for health insurance competency is more acute for the nearly
14 million people[2] who now buy individual health insurance on an insurance marketplace, enabled by the Affordable Care Act. These individuals
don't just need to understand how to use a health plan chosen for them;
they must choose a plan *and* use it wisely.

Noah was one of these individual health insurance buyers, without the
requisite expertise to feel confident about his selection. He hadn't expected
to need much expertise. Rather, he had expected the presentation of his

health insurance options to resemble what he might find on a typical online shopping site: a semi-customized recommendation based on his likely needs. "Other online businesses sort of prescribe options to you based on what your needs are, [like], 'if you're this kind of consumer, you're probably looking for this.'" He thought the health insurance marketplace website might explain, "This is good if you basically are a healthy 30-year-old that has no chronic illnesses." He hoped he would find a shortcut.

Instead, the options were not "clearly separated or sorted into categories." There were numerous variables that did not seem at all curated. "I guess it assumed you knew what you're looking for; it didn't really profile things." There was no beginner's guide. "It almost reminded me of plane tickets to get somewhere. It was like, 'here's what they cost, if you want to get from Portland to Miami.'" But Noah didn't think health insurance was anything like a plane ticket, which he saw as a utilitarian purchase to get from point A to point B. "Health insurance is supposed to be adapted to your life, I assume. I thought it would be a little bit more intuitive that way. Not to mention I didn't know what a deductible was." He couldn't weigh the choices without understanding what the words even meant.

Bella, a young woman who struggled to navigate her first health insurance purchase, described in Chapter 12, was not confident she understood what she had purchased. Did she have a deductible? She didn't think so. Copayments? She thought so but wasn't sure how much they were. Did she have coinsurance? Bella laughed and admitted, "Don't know what coinsurance means."

How can anyone shop for a product they don't fundamentally understand, much less use it effectively? Evaluating options and feeling confident in one's decision rest on a level of literacy most Americans don't have when it comes to health insurance. In one survey,[3] 96% of respondents could not correctly identify four out of four basic health insurance terms—including "deductible." Worse, unlike Noah, most people surveyed were overconfident in their knowledge, believing they knew more than they did. For example, only half the people surveyed could correctly define a deductible, but nearly three-quarters expressed confidence in their understanding of this term.

Researchers found similar results in a study of college students' health insurance literacy[4]—defined here as the ability to use health insurance effectively. Participants were tested for their knowledge of common health insurance terms and on their ability to calculate their costs in two hypothetical situations. This study also showed gaps in general knowledge of—and the ability to properly apply—health insurance concepts.

On average, participants correctly identified 15 of 20 terms, or 75%—not terrible. By category, though, only 2% could correctly identify all terminology related to plan options and just 18% correctly identified all cost-sharing terminology. One of the least well-understood terms was "coinsurance," which only 27% of students identified correctly.

Using these terms correctly proved even more challenging. Most (88%) could not correctly calculate their costs in both scenarios presented in the study. Half the respondents admitted they were confused about choosing or using their health plan, and one-quarter said their confusion had stopped or delayed them from getting medical care.

Before the assessment, students had felt capable in this arena, with most respondents (64%) expressing confidence in their knowledge. After being tested, though, less than half (41%) maintained that confidence. Those who gave themselves higher marks for health insurance vocabulary knowledge did fare better; not only did they identify more terms correctly, they were also better at figuring out their financial responsibility accurately in the two scenarios. That finding suggests that health insurance literacy leads to more accurate interpretations of, and greater ability to use, health benefits.

THE COST OF HEALTH INSURANCE ILLITERACY

Given America's immensely complex health care system, it's no wonder we have high rates of health insurance illiteracy. An Accenture study showed that 52% of Americans had low health-system literacy.[5] "There is a profound amount of confusion among both consumers as well as people who are supposed to be the purported experts," Ann Sweeney told me. Founder of Acadia Consulting, a human resources consulting firm, she has overseen countless health insurance open enrollment processes.

Lois Mills, an insurance broker who helps businesses find and buy health insurance for employees, agreed that consumers are confused. "[Employees] don't really know how to begin to navigate it, to evaluate it."

Health insurance illiteracy has concrete economic implications: it wastes money. The same Accenture study[6] estimated that consumer health insurance illiteracy costs $4 billion a year, up to three-quarters of which could be waste. Accenture blames impenetrable jargon, convoluted rules, and lack of clarity over how to access benefits. Confused consumers, then, clog customer service lines to seek clarification or to argue after they find that something they expected to be covered was not. Health plans must invest in staff and systems to manage those calls, spending which could theoretically be reduced if confusion were lessened. To their credit, Accenture's prescription is not to educate consumers better but rather to call for insurers to simplify their processes and language.

Health insurance illiteracy also hits individuals' pocketbooks. People who are less health insurance literate spend more than they need to, essentially over-buying coverage. Researchers studied a scenario in which one health plan option would cost more no matter what services the consumer used.[7] In this menu of options, there was an objectively right answer. Still, people chose the most costly plan with no additional benefit, apparently—though erroneously—thinking they could reduce financial exposure by paying more each month. For example, employees would have to pay more than $500 in annual premiums to lower their deductible from $1,000 to $750. No matter how much health care spending one could have, under no circumstances would it make sense to pay $500 more per year to save $250.

These suboptimal decisions were inequitably distributed.[8] Employees earning less than $40,000 per year were much more likely to choose the unnecessarily expensive plans, even though they were less able to absorb those expenses than their better-compensated colleagues. Employees who were likely to need more health care services and have higher medical expenses—female and older employees and those with chronic medical conditions—were also more likely to choose the unduly expensive plans. In the study, nearly a quarter of employees switched plans for modest improvements, but lower-income employees were less likely to switch plans or to switch into the most economically favorable plan if they did.

Whatever the source of consumer miscalculation—confusion, anxiety, or carelessness—it is no one's primary job to help consumers make good choices. Health plans have a perverse incentive *not* to help consumers avoid these miscalculations. That is not to say they actively don't want to help consumers, but their economic interests may be better served by consumer ignorance. When consumers spend more on health coverage than they need, insurers make more money in premiums.

Employers may not want employees to squander money or to be dissatisfied with the value of their health benefits. And employers have no reason to encourage employees to over-buy health insurance. But employers' direct interest is in overall benefit costs, not any one individual's spending, and it may not be against their immediate or direct interests if employees do overspend. Whether these incentives dominate decisions or hover unconsciously in the background, it is safe to say that employees lose out more than their employers when they over-pay for insurance.

"They present as helpless," Ann Sweeney told me of employees during health insurance open enrollment. "There's too much information being presented and being presented in a manner that's too confusing for them to make an accurate assessment." Overwhelmed employees struggle to make informed choices.

Sweeney has worked with start-ups and larger technical organizations, full of highly educated professionals who still struggled to understand health insurance information as presented to them. Nationally, nearly half of low-health-system-literate respondents held college and/or graduate degrees, and virtually all (97%) had high school diplomas.[9] Thus, health insurance confusion has more to do with cultural norms and lack of health-system knowledge than overall education, Sweeney said. "[People] haven't been taught to ask questions about their health care." She found that people "want someone to make the decision for them. I have had scores of people come to me and say 'can you just choose for me?' These are people with PhDs. . . . What chance does the average person have to be able to make an informed decision?"

CONFUSING BY DESIGN

George, a New York finance professional introduced in Chapter 6, theorized that insurers' profit motive explains the confusion. "A lot of this stuff is made confusing intentionally, maybe for two reasons. One is for the insurer to protect itself by confusing what gets covered and what doesn't, but separately, to entice people or to scare people into selecting the most expensive plan."

Sweeney shared George's question about insurers' intentions. "I am always struck by how non-straightforward a lot of information is presented to people who are supposed to be making an informed decision about their health care." During open enrollment periods, Sweeney advocated for information to be presented to employees in clear and digestible form. She rarely, if ever, saw that happen, whether because health plans lose perspective on plain language or because "there's some deliberateness around crafting obfuscation because it will result in a sustained state of consumer ignorance." Consumer ignorance favors health insurers because "people don't know even what to ask."

Accenture's study suggests reducing confusion could benefit health insurers directly because less confusion could lead to administrative efficiencies and associated savings. But simplification is hard to achieve—likely requiring investment—and any savings would be hard to realize. Even if less confusion resulted in fewer calls and a smaller number of customer service staff needed, cutting or redeploying staff is difficult. Further, confusion may inadvertently lead to increased insurance revenues when people buy more coverage than they need. Reducing confusion, therefore, could lead people to buy more appropriate levels of coverage and decrease health plan revenues. Any cost savings from administrative simplification would need to offset those lost revenues for insurers. The power of financial incentives, particularly the fear of jeopardizing revenue, explains a lot about why change is slow to come to the health insurance industry.

ILLITERACY LEADS TO AVOIDANCE

Health insurance illiteracy also has human costs. People avoid using health benefits—postponing or avoiding needed care—because they fear unknown costs. This fear sometimes hinders good decision-making.

As discussed in Chapter 8, Amanda avoided the emergency room during acute appendicitis because she did not realize emergency care would be covered. Similarly, fear of unknown costs deterred Hannah from going to the hospital when she was hit by a car while riding her bike. "I was in shock, so I thought I was okay and denied going in the ambulance to a hospital." In the moment, the hospital felt like "a big ordeal" that wasn't necessary, and she worried it would be costly. She later discovered she had suffered a concussion and what developed into long-term chronic neck pain. Letting concern over cost interfere with getting the care she needed? "That's something I regret."

The relationship between health insurance literacy and rates of delaying or foregoing care is clear. One-third[10] of people had delayed or foregone care because of cost; people with lower health insurance literacy reported higher rates of avoiding care. This phenomenon affects some groups more than others, exacerbating health disparities between ethnic groups. The Urban Institute's Health Policy Center[11] found lower confidence in one's health insurance literacy among non-whites compared to whites.

Even for otherwise privileged consumers, health insurance illiteracy creates obstacles. Dave reflected on the cost of health insurance illiteracy, when he tried to fight his health plan's decision to cut off his mental health benefits—described in Chapter 3—because they questioned the medical necessity of his psychotherapy. He felt the ruling was inconsistent with mental health parity laws. "Contesting it was like arguing your own case in court. The burden of proof used terminology and standards, and those words that you don't have access to." The energy he deployed was fruitless; the health plan said he was too late to contest their initial decision.

For Lillian, a part-time nurse and Medicare enrollee, health insurance confusion created barriers to using benefits. "I don't find it ever not frustrating dealing with insurance stuff. And I think, 'I know terminology. I know what the heck they're talking about,' and then I don't know what they're talking about. I think I know what I'm doing and I just still can't figure it all out. It's so convoluted."

Though generally satisfied with Medicare, Lillian blamed the public nature of the program for undue confusion. "All of it has certain government touches to it; that's probably why we get volumes and volumes of literature and just so much of the different competing supplemental insurance plans that are out there. They just sort of overwhelm you with information." In Lillian's view, the federal agency that provides nearly all Americans 65 and over with health insurance—and is trying to protect these consumers and make sure they have what they need to make informed decisions—inadvertently contributes to health insurance confusion.

IMPROVING CONSUMER HEALTH INSURANCE LITERACY

Health insurance illiteracy is not just a function of consumer education or capabilities; it reflects a series of practices that institutions—mainly health plans—employ, deliberately or inadvertently keeping consumers confused. Consumers should be able to expect better.

Health care—and insurance in particular—runs on jargon, defined as "technical terminology or characteristic idiom of a special activity or group often employed with a tacit assumption of common understanding."[12] Once people have mastered that language, they seem to lose sight of how hard it was to learn originally. Insiders tend to abuse that "tacit assumption of common understanding." As a health insurance executive once said on a panel we shared at a health care consumer engagement conference, "It's hard to read the label from inside the jar." In other words, being immersed in the terminology makes it hard to know how confusing it is for others.

Health plans should start with how consumers receive information, rather than with how they want or know how to deliver it. When developing consumer communications, insurers should start with questions like: What do consumers know and understand? What confuses consumers? How does it feel to navigate health insurance from a consumer's point of view?

Helen Osborne, who trains organizations on health literacy and plain-language writing, worries about leaders who don't invest in these principles. "It's pretty easy to make a compelling case about why this matters," Osborne said, especially with the people doing everyday communications work. But those who choose not to attend her seminars "are probably the ones making the big decisions anyway, and the most influential ones." Too often, she has found "the people who needed to hear it," that is, the people with power and influence in organizations, "didn't prioritize it."

Health insurance concepts can be complex, and health plans could do more to lessen confusion. "Health care, honestly, has lagged way behind," Osborne said of the industry's ability to convey clear messages. "Marketing can do it well. Journalism can do it well. They know how to be clear and succinct." Why not in health care? More health plans, for example, could elevate a role for consumer marketers and experts in consumer communications—already in place at some health plans—to reshape the voice of the plan with the expertise Osborne referenced.

"It takes a team to write a readable document," she said. "Your team needs to include your subject matter experts. It also needs to include someone who's skilled and savvy in plain-language writing, and an unceasing advocate for the reader." The team must, she said, "include those who represent the audience."

Complexity is not the sole purview of the plans; regulators often make matters worse in pursuit of transparency and disclosure to protect consumers. As Lillian noted about the apparent government influence on Medicare communications, regulators play a significant role in perpetuating and cementing sometimes impenetrable jargon.

When I led the marketing department of a small health plan, my team produced advertising and website content, as well as member handbooks, ID cards, health information, and required notices. In serving low- and moderate-income members on subsidized insurance programs, state contracts and Medicaid regulations governed our work. Medicaid required all health plan member communications to be written at a 6th-grade reading level to ensure that members—often low-literacy or non-native-English speakers—could understand important information about their rights to access health care services. We developed an extensive review process and used a standard measurement tool that calculates what grade the average reader would need to have completed to understand the document. If that measure came back too high, we would revise the document until it was in an acceptable range, though we never reached 6th-grade.

We learned and applied tips: Simplify word choices. Avoid complex sentence structures. Avoid the passive voice (as in, replace "Mistakes were made" with "We made mistakes"). Keep documents as short as possible. We even hired a full-time editor who had his own bag of tricks for simplifying language. Consumers can't demand that health plans hire for specific roles or adopt certain processes, but they can make complaints and raise questions, nudging plans to improve communications by expressing confusion and dissatisfaction.

I remember one document we worked on—maybe a letter—that was particularly tricky; we were having little luck getting the document lower than a 12th-grade reading level. As an experiment, we deleted the state's required language and re-measured. It dropped to an 8th-grade reading level! Of course, we had to keep that language in the document, but we had discovered the tangible cost of government regulation in terms of readability. That language aims to protect consumers by fully informing them, but often makes it virtually impossible for the average person to comprehend. In the end, the effort to protect consumers can obscure the knowledge it's meant to confer.

In a perfect world, health plans and insurance regulators would commit to improving health insurance literacy and measure such improvements through consumers' eyes, not their own. They would create review processes that included end-user feedback and then act on that feedback. They would favor true clarity over bureaucratic compliance and evolve dynamically rather than layer requirement upon crusty-old legacy requirement.

It would benefit consumers if health plans would take some of my advice. But we should not wait passively for a complex, heavily regulated industry to change itself or for the industry's regulators to trade bureaucratic approaches for market-worthy standards. Although I assign a greater share of responsibility for health insurance literacy to the industry, there are things consumers can and should do to help themselves navigate this lingo.

1.   Act like you're spending your own money

In the study of college student insurance literacy,[13] students who paid their own premiums scored better on the insurance vocabulary test than those whose parents paid it or those who had university subsidies to cover those costs.

Most Americans *are* paying, at least in part, for our health care, whether we realize it or not. It's obvious when we take out a credit card to pay a copayment at the doctor's office or write a check to pay monthly premiums. Fewer people are as attuned to the monthly contribution their employer might take directly out of their paycheck; even people who know they pay part of their health insurance premium rarely know the exact amount of the automatic deduction.

Lois Mills, the insurance broker who has decades of experience helping employees choosing and using health insurance, explained that people tend to fixate on their direct out-of-pocket costs. "It's like your electric— you pay your bill (each month), but if every time (you turned on the light) you had to pay $2, you'd think about it more." People notice the value of their health insurance, she said, when they get COBRA, which allows employees to buy their employer's health plan without any employer contribution for 18 months after they leave that employer. Paying full price for their employer benefits gives most people sticker shock, according to Mills, but it should also underscore the economic value employers contribute to employees via health benefits.

Indirectly, though, even people with generous health benefits through their employer should banish the notion that they "get it for free." Employers routinely calculate benefits into the total compensation. That means your employer thinks of your health benefits as part of what they pay you. In fact, many organizations offset lower pay scales with more generous benefits. Health benefits are an extension of your paycheck in your employer's mind; you should recognize this benefit as part of your compensation and treat it accordingly. The average benefit cost is approximately 32% of total compensation.[14] A 2018 report showed the average employer-sponsored health insurance preferred provider organization (PPO) plan for a family of four cost more than $28,000 and employers paid approximately 56% of the cost.[15] Finally, for any American who pays taxes, you are contributing to your future Medicare costs. Most Medicare enrollees worked for decades to qualify for such benefits, paying in a little bit each paycheck they received.

So, treat your health insurance benefits like you're paying for them. In most cases, that's at least partly true.

2.   Ask more questions

Because I have an allergy to peppers—bell peppers, chili, and all derivatives—going out to eat can be dicey for me. I love to eat out so I do it anyway. I have learned to read menus carefully, disclose my allergy, ask many questions, and trust my instinct if a server doesn't seem to be listening closely enough to understand my allergy. If my food arrives with any red hue or if it makes the back of my throat burn, I escalate. This process can be exhausting, but my health is at stake.

Health care consumers should similarly invest in the process to interrogate their health benefits. What is covered? What will it cost? What does this word mean? How does this concept relate to my access to care and my costs? Asking these kinds of questions—until you genuinely feel confident that you understand—flows from behaving as if you pay for your own health care, even if an employer or the government or your parents or your spouse pay for all or part of your coverage.

Whom should you ask? Call the health plan customer service line, or ask your doctor's office. If you have employer-based coverage, ask your human resources department. If not, call the agency that oversees the process, like the state or federal exchange, Medicare, or Medicaid. For publicly funded insurance programs, there are often navigators, helpers, or other nonprofit organizations funded—or committed—to helping consumers navigate the process.

If you don't wear an item of clothing you buy, even if you got a good deal, you've paid too much. Similarly, if you can't use your health insurance because you don't understand how it works or what the words even mean, you're potentially leaving value on the table.

3.   Learn the basic terminology

Health insurance lingo is not fixed; it has evolved and will continue to evolve. Health plans will likely introduce new designs and new types of cost-sharing. As new terms arise, consumers will need to adjust and evolve. Still, it's worth mastering some basic terms in current use.

Most people know that copayments are the fees you pay when you get a health care service[16] and premiums are the amount you pay for your health insurance each month,[17] but far and away the most confusing term seems to be "coinsurance."

What the heck is coinsurance?

Coinsurance is a percentage of health care costs you have to pay, with the insurance company paying the rest. Increasingly common, coinsurance accounts for almost one-third of consumer cost-sharing. Spending on coinsurance rose faster (67% growth) than overall cost-sharing (54%) between 2006 and 2016.[18]

Typically, coinsurance kicks in after you've satisfied your deductible and you have to pay a share of health care charges. Like co-parenting, where people share child-rearing responsibilities, coinsurance is like sharing financial responsibility for your medical expenses with your insurance company.

The tricky thing about coinsurance is that it is typically a percentage of the health care charges, which can be nearly impossible to find, as discussed in Chapter 5. One health plan defines "coinsurance" as "a percentage of the amount *we allow to be charged*."[19] What do they allow to be charged? I called this plan to see how I might get information on the allowed charges. Not surprisingly, the answer was "it depends." There was no centralized, publicly available list of charges. Anticipating and accurately calculating coinsurance might be impossible. Thus, understanding what the word coinsurance means is an important start but that alone won't tell you what coinsurance may cost you.

Here are nine other terms, from the college-student survey,[20] that often confuse people:

1. **Deductible:** "The amount you pay for covered health care services before your insurance plan starts to pay"[21]

2. **Out-of-pocket maximum:** "The most you have to pay for covered services in a plan year" in deductibles, copayments, and coinsurance (not including premiums); after you've paid this maximum amount, the health plan should pay 100% of costs of covered services[22]

3. **Formulary:** A list of prescription drugs covered by a prescription drug or other insurance plan (also called a drug list)[23]

4. **Annual limit:** A cap on the benefits an insurance company will pay in a year, sometimes placed on dollar amounts of covered services or a number of visits of a particular service (usually consumers have to pay all the costs of services beyond the insurance company's cap)[24]

5. **Prior authorization:** A health plan's approval that may be required before you get a service or fill a prescription[25]

6. **HMO (Health Maintenance Organization):** "A type of health insurance plan that usually limits coverage to care from doctors who work for or contract with the HMO"[26]

7. **HRA (Health Reimbursement Account or Arrangement):** Employer-funded and -owned accounts out of which employees are reimbursed tax-free for qualified medical expenses up to a fixed dollar amount per year; unused amounts may be rolled over to be used in subsequent years[27]

8. **HSA (Health Savings Account):** A savings account—offered by an insurer or a financial institution—into which consumers in high-deductible health plans can set aside a limited amount of pre-tax money to pay for qualified medical expenses[28]

9. **FSA (Flexible Spending Account or Arrangement):** An arrangement through an employer that allows consumers to pay many out-of-pocket medical expenses with tax-free dollars; consumers typically decide how much to put into an FSA up to a limit set by the employer[29]

Learning this terminology will not, by itself, make you health insurance literate or confident in your understanding of your benefits and their costs, but it's a start. By understanding the vocabulary, you can at least be more confident in asking relevant questions. And studies show that people with more facility with the vocabulary make better, more economically beneficial decisions.

DEMAND THAT HEALTH CARE GET OUT OF ITS JAR

Health care is complicated. In particular, health insurance language is unique, not intuitive, and hard to learn. The stakes are high, so regulators take great pains to try to protect consumers. Health plans focus heavily on complying with those regulatory requirements. They're stuck inside the jar. With an ever-intensifying focus on consumerism in health care, they might start to realize they're inside the jar but not necessarily be set up to get themselves out. Our job, as consumers, is to knock on that jar. Look at it critically. Ask the questions and point to what makes no sense. Demand clarity and transparency. Keep knocking. It's the only way short of learning the whole language yourself to bring about change.

12

It's No Kayak

Why choosing health insurance is so hard for humans

There is no joy in choosing a health insurance plan. "It's about as much fun as estate planning, deciding a living will, who's going to take your kids if you both die and, decisions like that," said Dave, a 50-year-old with a wife and children. "You're dealing with an opaque system that doesn't leave you with very much choice, and the choices presented to you don't correlate very well to the outcomes."

Dave's feelings about health insurance purchasing are well founded. Health insurance products are difficult to understand. The language involved is indeed opaque, as discussed in Chapter 11. Comparing options can be confusing; if you don't understand the terminology that describes one plan, it's very difficult to effectively compare across plans. If you have too many options, you may feel it's impossible to decipher meaningful differences; too few, and it can be hard to find the right fit.

Even when choosing between limited employer-offered options, many consumers feel overwhelmed. Dave did not feel confident about his ability to accurately anticipate the risks health insurance is designed to mitigate. "You don't have much guidance. If you buy insurance for your house, in a short conversation, you can end up with a number which seems right, which seems sufficient. And then you're out of there. But with health care, even these things that are routine leave you wondering."

Jason, a 35-year-old chief technology officer at a start-up that doesn't offer health benefits, said of buying health insurance on the federal marketplace, "It's the most confusing system. I have a Harvard education and it's completely incomprehensible." On the cusp of open enrollment when we spoke, he had yet to start exploring options. "I don't want that soul-sucking adventure to start until it *has* to start."

For people with health insurance, status quo bias[1]—or inertia—tends to tip the scales for whatever plan they're on. But when someone is new to the insurance market or forced to choose a new option, the process can be overwhelming. Simply put, choosing health insurance is hard—confusing and sometimes scary. To effectively navigate insurance choices, people must anticipate their future risks and needs, identify their preferences, and ultimately make sometimes difficult trade-offs.

FACING COMPLEXITY

Many components can factor into health plan selection—access to providers, coverage of specific services or medications, administrative hurdles of accessing benefits, customer service and quality ratings, and most important for many people, cost.

Costs are not always easy to discern, judge, or compare. Not only are they comprised of many different elements—monthly premiums, copayments, coinsurance, deductibles—but those elements apply differently to everyone. Costs depend on so many factors—prescription drugs, providers, site of service, to name a few. Some factors may be known or knowable, while others involve assessment of probability, preference, and risk tolerance.

When choosing health insurance each year, Tara tries to anticipate what services she, her husband, and her baby might use over the course of the year. "We consider our options and do a post-analysis on what we could predict that we will need. And then, we consider affordability versus level of care." Affordability can be calculated in a variety of ways; how does Tara think about it? "We do an annual monetary expense to see through the course of the year under this insurance plan, what could we estimate that we would need to be spending."

A motivated and educated consumer, Louisa also tries to project her total health care costs for the year, calculating premiums plus copayments for the services she anticipates her family will use. She guesses what the best- and worst-case scenarios might be. "If we're risk averse, we might go on the one that—if things go worse—is going still end up with us being in a decent shape. That's how we originally did it."

The structure of cost-sharing components like copayments and coinsurance can matter nearly as much as the total amounts consumers need to pay. For example, in Chapter 11, insurance broker Lois Mills described how much people notice when copayments increase for primary care visits. Kevin McDevitt, former IT implementation manager at the Massachusetts Health Connector, the state's health insurance marketplace, confirmed that a Massachusetts Connector survey showed PCP copayments were a top concern for consumers.

In addition to sorting out the optimal mix of premiums and out-of-pocket costs components, consumers must also attend to aspects of their current treatment, including their physician and medication costs. Joseph Newhouse, PhD, professor of health policy at Harvard University, noted that finding the right health plan is not easy for consumers in this regard. "It's very hard to get information about how broad the specialist network is," he explained. He described how virtually all primary care providers, at least in the Boston area, participate in all the major plans, but specialists do not. "The specialist networks are much more limited, and most people don't care about that until they need the specialist. And you don't know which one you might need," he explained. "So defaulting to the primary care doc, I think that's probably the most you could do unless you know you want a specialist and if you're on a non-generic drug. Then those questions certainly matter."

For some consumers, access to specific doctors or specific services are most important, even if it means paying more for other things. Simone chose her family's plan around specific providers. "I want to make sure that the pediatrician that I like is covered on my plan. I want to make sure that the hospitals that I like are covered on my plan." Noah narrowed down his health insurance choices based on his therapist, whose fees he couldn't afford without insurance. When the therapist urged Noah not to sign up for Medicaid if he qualified because of the administrative hassles and delays in the therapist's reimbursement, Noah chose the plan the therapist specifically recommended.

Other consumers prioritize health plan brand or reputation, often as a proxy for plans that may be easier to deal with. J.J. told me she didn't think of herself as brand oriented, but she said, "I am more likely to go with something that isn't going to have any surprises." When she was younger, she would have opted for the least expensive option, but then she had a devastating experience: she had a severely disabled daughter who had died many years before we met. Insurance battles on her daughter's behalf gave J.J. an appreciation for health plan reliability, and she used brand reputation as a proxy for that less concrete measure.

Intertwined with brand is perception of quality, which can be hard to discern, as discussed in Chapter 9. I asked Kevin McDevitt whether quality ratings had resonance for consumers shopping for health insurance in Massachusetts. "I think that's a really hard thing to define," he said.

Virtually all Massachusetts health plans have high ratings from accrediting bodies; without quality-rating variability, it's difficult to choose a plan based on quality. Even in geographies where there are more meaningful differences between higher- and lower-rated plans, quality ratings are based largely on how good participating providers are and on broad-brush customer satisfaction ratings. Though based on detailed surveys, results are boiled down so much that it can be hard to tell how much bureaucratic hassle there is for plan members or how much value the plan delivers.

DIFFICULT TRADE-OFFS

The core decisions in health plan purchasing require making trade-offs between these elements, often focusing specifically on various cost elements. Consumers try to predict their future needs and identify their tolerance for risk. Like squeezing air from one side of a balloon to another, the higher the deductible, typically, the lower the monthly premium. People paying higher premiums are effectively prepaying the cost of any health care services they may need in that year. If they need more care than they have prepaid, the insurance company bears the financial risk and may lose money on that member.

Conversely, people who opt to pay less out of pocket in exchange for a higher deductible take on some of that risk themselves. If they can avoid care, they haven't paid for services they didn't need. If they do need services, they'll pay the first $1,000, $2,000, or even $8,000 of those bills—whatever the amount of the deductible. Not everyone chooses to take this greater level of financial risk based on an informed assessment of likely limited need. Rather, for many, choosing a high-deductible health plan is based on financial necessity and a prayer. If you cannot afford a higher premium, you have to hope you won't need to pay for services under the deductible.

Consumers adopt a range of strategies for balancing up-front costs with future out-of-pocket risks. Jason tried to weed out plans by finding the plan with the best coverage for his asthma medication—a generic drug—but no plan covered it. Though it was developed in the 1970s and he figured out it costs $6 to make, Jason paid $250 per prescription. "I don't know why it's not covered. It completely baffles me."

Absent a preference based on medication coverage, he opted for the lowest premium, reasoning that at least his monthly cost is a certainty. "I basically look for the cheapest amount that I'm required to pay and then I endeavor to pay nothing on top of that." His trade-off is clear: by opting for lower-premium plans, he usually has such a high deductible that he never meets it. "It's just going to be me paying for everything." To minimize his out-of-pocket costs, Jason just tries to avoid health care altogether.

Brooke, a young adult buying health insurance on her own for the first time, figured out how to visualize insurance trade-offs by entering different variables into the insurance marketplace website, which served up different options in response. "When I refresh the page and put in different options, I found one that was $250 a month and I don't have a deductible on this one but my copays are still a little bit higher, especially for specialists." She could see that some of the plans were clearly the wrong choice: "Some of the most expensive ones that I looked at were like $300 to $400 a month, but still had a huge deductible in the thousands, like $5,000 to $7,000 deductible, and the copays were not any cheaper. Who would purchase this plan?"

As clever as she was in her shopping process, Brooke still struggled to project her out-of-pocket costs. She said, "I kind of knew what a deductible was because I have car insurance but I didn't know what that would apply towards in terms of health care." Understanding the concept of a deductible did not help her grasp the practicalities of what things would cost if she used her benefits. "Say I go to the doctor for a sinus infection. It's not a physical, so I know I'm paying my copay when I go. But what would my deductible be?" Would the antibiotic she was prescribed count toward her deductible? Would the visit itself count? Do copayments count? She had no idea how the deductible worked in reality.

Brooke faced another challenge common to new health insurance shoppers: young and healthy, Brooke didn't have any experience to inform her choice. "I have only been to my doctors once in the past two years. I don't need anything else besides a well-visit. I've never needed medicine." The health insurance shopping process didn't give her enough information to know for sure what her true financial liability could be. Two years later, she said, "I still have no idea."

Like any health plan shopper, Brooke needed to assess probabilities: how likely was it that she would incur different kinds of costs in the next year? Some consumers are willing to go to great lengths to wrangle these probabilities, but even with an investment of energy, Dave sensed he lacks the power to make effective choices. "There are a few different options. But, even though the numbers exist out there for it to be knowable which one is going to be the best fit for you, you're left making a decision based on very difficult-to-ascertain rules."

Dave went on, "To figure out the best health plan, it's hard enough to guess what's going to happen in the next year, but it is possible to make some good assumptions." Even though it might be possible to make educated assumptions, the process of estimating likely utilization and calculating the cost of different scenarios, according to Dave, "sucks. It takes a lot of hours and involves a lot of uncertainty." Putting in more time and effort might save Dave money, but he felt that "if you see diminishing returns you have to cut and decide, but it shouldn't have to be that way. Let me just say, it's not Kayak. And purchasing health care could be more like that." The streamlined, consumer-grade technology that transformed the travel industry could similarly improve the health insurance selection process. "You could commoditize these coverages, services based on your prior use to see what the cost structure would be like according to different levels and needs."

THERE MAY BE A RIGHT ANSWER, BUT HUMANS AREN'T NECESSARILY SUITED TO FIND IT

Most consumer decisions do not have an objectively "right answer"—the consumer's preferences typically matter most. This is often the case in health insurance. "Usually, it's a judgment call," said Tal Gross, PhD, associate professor at Boston University's Questrom School of Business.

But sometimes, there is an objectively better health insurance option that consumers often miss, like in the study described in Chapter 11, where consumers consistently make the wrong choice.[2] Gross explained it this way: "You have two plans. They are all the same network, all the same benefits. The difference between the two plans is just the premium and cost-sharing. You can do the math and in this case, one always dominates the other." Gross said, "You should just go with the one plan over the other. And people make the wrong choice."

Even when there is a right answer or a clearly better, higher-value choice, it may be exceedingly difficult for people to figure that out. "In some cases, there's a right answer," Gross said, "but you have to be a computer to figure it out. In other cases, there is a right answer but you need to know what your degree of risk aversion is. It gets a little tricky."

"People don't handle uncertainty very well, and they don't handle probabilities well," Professor Newhouse explained. For example, loss aversion tends to cloud rationality in insurance purchasing, which may lead people to buy more coverage than is likely to be necessary.[3] "We know what kind of mistakes people make. Insurance is a very complicated product, but it's about a risky situation, so it's not surprising that many people make mistakes."

CLOSER TO KAYAK

When I was around Brooke's age, I worked on a project to develop a marketing plan for a start-up that was going to sell individual health insurance policies directly to consumers—online. The year was 1999, and shopping online for health insurance was completely new. I interviewed individual health insurance consumers about their experiences with health insurance and learned that people dreaded the process so much that it was like receiving notice of an impending IRS audit. These consumers described having to call around to different health plans in their area, one by one, and ask for plan costs and information. They would then have to lay out the options—if they could even find more than one available carrier—and compare them. When I say "lay out the options," I mean spread out printed plan documents side by side—maybe on the kitchen table—and manually analyze differences between plans, calculate likely total costs, and then pick a plan.

Shopping for health insurance today is a lot more like Kayak or another airfare comparison tool than it used to be. But the tools consumers can use to compare and purchase health insurance still have room for improvement.

"I tried to do research on my own," said Gregg, an individual health insurance buyer. "I went online and it was just so utterly confusing and there were so many possibilities that I just felt like there was no way I could figure out the details of these plans."

Sandra, an independent consultant, described her experience shopping for family coverage on the insurance marketplace after her husband left his corporate job. She had to repeatedly answer the same questions to reclaim an account she had set up a year before but not used since. Each response she gave would generate a new tree of questions. It felt like a comedy of errors, but "we did get there."

Megan, the graduate student introduced in Chapter 7 who wished she understood health insurance better, had a more positive online shopping experience. "I was able to compare side by side in a pretty useful way," but the experience was still challenging: "I didn't know what everything meant. I think more like 'hover over this' and it says a definition, would have been useful." She had to do an online search for a lot of terms she could not get definitions for on the insurance site. "And then, the stuff I wasn't too embarrassed to ask . . . I've asked my parents."

Louisa's annual process to evaluate her husband's employer-sponsored benefits involved weighing trade-offs with the help of an online tool provided by the employer. "At work, they give you a bunch of pamphlets and originally there was a tool online and we went through and did all the cost benefit [analysis] and picked a plan," she explained. "But that turned out to be wrong because they were such a pain in the ass to work with." They switched plans in a subsequent year to one reported to have better customer service, even though it cost more. "They've gone up in price but we've stayed with them," she said. The online tool hadn't accounted for the less-tangible hassle factor.

"It's easy to give up," acknowledged Kevin McDevitt. Despite constant improvements to the health insurance shopping process and close attention to the user experience on the insurance marketplaces, the way choices are presented needs improvement, he said. "The information is not easy to understand. I feel like we're still kind of at square one. We don't have great tools to help people and I'm not aware that anyone else really does."

His approach to improving the online insurance shopping experience at the Massachusetts marketplace—and mitigating choice overload—was to figure out what matters most to consumers and present those elements to people in a clear way. "There's a lot of jargony terms. There's a lot of moving parts." The priority needs to be "trying to make that as simple as possible using simple language in the displays, making it as clear as possible about what they're supposed to do on each page."

When he and I spoke in 2017, the Massachusetts marketplace had eight different filters in the plan display, which didn't fit in one screen. Users would have to scroll down to see them all, which people just don't do. McDevitt worked on limiting the amount of information presented to consumers by trimming the number of filters, reserving website real estate for those elements that consumers cared about the most. "Price and provider network are far and away the two biggest components that go into purchasing a health insurance plan," McDevitt explained. Those would be front and center, with less distraction from less important categories. The filters would all be there for consumers who chose to drill down into those details, just like you might find on "Zappos or one of those very consumer-friendly sites." It's good news for consumers that health insurance marketplaces are moving toward these consumer-grade models.

CHOICE ARCHITECTURE

Even though technology can help present choices more efficiently, it can't deliver the right number of choices. That's personal.

Some consumers feel overloaded by too many choices, and evidence suggests having more choices does not necessarily improve the quality of decisions.[4] For example, after Sandra got through the circuitous and repetitive questions to recover her online account on the state's health insurance marketplace, the representative who was helping her offered 40 different plans. Based on Sandra's interest in good prescription drug coverage and a preference for a known health plan brand, they whittled the list to a more manageable and comparable assortment.

Even as many people feel overwhelmed by the number of health plan options, some people want *more* choice. In her book *Who Killed Health*

Care,[5] Regina Herzlinger of the Harvard Business School advocates for more health insurance options to meet a broader array of consumer needs and preferences. A wider health plan selection could also theoretically help contain health costs and improve quality if adoption of higher-value plans nudged the market toward greater overall value.

Ralph wished for more options when shopping for Medicare plans. He had six plans available, but not all matched his criteria. "I had to make compromises."

Brooke also wished she had more choices, because she didn't like any of the available plans. "When I went on Healthcare.gov this year, all of my options were [from one company]. And I know they're not the only insurance provider out there. But that's all it gave me." Unsatisfied, her biggest complaint was with the trade-offs she had to make between extremely high deductibles for lower premiums or very high premiums for no deductible. "I feel like I was choosing the lesser of two evils."

Brooke wasn't accustomed to such limited shopping experiences. "I didn't even know if I could look elsewhere or where to look if I could. If you shop for car insurance or life insurance, you can just Google search 'car insurance,' and you can get a quote from 50 different companies and choose which one has the best coverage for the best price." Her health insurance experience felt completely different. "I was stuck just going to one place. It's like, 'You can either go to Walmart or you can go to Walmart.' You can't go to Target or Costco and price shop between these different companies. You literally just have one option. That's kind of what I would like to see change, because I feel like that would probably drive cost down, if there's more to choose from and more competition."

MISERY LOVES COMPANY

Some consumers don't even try to tackle health insurance purchasing on their own. They seek professional help from insurance agents.

Theo described his confusion with the process. "It's inscrutable. I don't understand the plan. Plus, I don't know which plans have better track records, which have worse track records. Actually, you have secret language which makes the plan difficult." To overcome this confusion, Theo used an insurance agent because, as he said, "God knows, I could not figure this out by myself." The agent showed him how he could trade a narrower selection of doctors for slightly smaller premiums or pay about $50 more per month for more flexibility.

Hazel took the same approach to mitigate her confusion. As discussed in Chapter 4, Hazel never considered shopping alone. "I wouldn't even know where to begin," she said, admitting to stumbling on some health insurance terms, like Theo and the consumers described in Chapter 11.

"There are some confusing terms in there that I'm sure aren't that big of a deal if you take the time to figure them out."

Her husband's company was switching plans around the time one of Hazel's employees asked about getting health benefits through the small business. Hazel called on an agent to help her sort out whether her family would be better off if Hazel bought a small group plan to cover the employees and her family or if they should stick with her husband's plan.

Agents are common in her area, and she was inclined to believe that the people who do it all the time could help her make sense of the process and choose better plans. "I figured if I could just have someone who knew what they were talking about, they could advise me. And I, kind of in general, trust people to do what they know." She added, "I do have this slight suspicion that it's like taxes, if you don't know what you're doing, you're not going to get a good deal." She did not research plans on her own but reviewed the agent's recommendations and picked one.

When it came time to use her benefits and understand what was covered and what was subject to the deductible, she acknowledged, "That stuff is never that clear to me. I know it's all written right there, but that's why I get agents. It's always kind of a mystery to me."

BUT WHAT SHOULD I DO?

Because of my professional experience working for a health plan, people often ask me to help them sort out health insurance as they transition jobs, lose COBRA, or arrive in the United States from overseas.

"What should I do," people ask, even people with incredible professional achievements and great intellect. Even extremely competent people often start at square one with navigating health insurance. No one is immune from feeling completely lost.

When people ask me for help, I introduce them to the ACA marketplace and accompany them as much as I can on their selection process, starting with a few questions:

1. **Providers**: Do you have a doctor or set of doctors you care about? Is there a hospital you're committed to having access to? I suggest we first look at which health plans include those providers in their networks.

2. **Medications**: Do you take any prescriptions? If so, what tier are those drugs on, and what would the copayment be on different plans? Does the drug require prior authorization? If so, you may be able to get it, but it is not guaranteed and it may involve some hassle. Jason had tried to anchor his selection on his asthma medication, but no plan

covered it, so it did not help narrow his choices and he had to start from scratch.

3. **Preferences**: Would you rather pay more for certainty or take the risk of paying out of pocket under a deductible for services you need? Without getting too personal, I ask, how healthy are you? What do you expect your needs to be?

I tested my approach with Harvard's Professor Newhouse to see how I might improve my guidance to colleagues. He didn't have anything to add, given the degree of uncertainty we all face in predicting our future health care needs. My simple framework, apparently, isn't missing much.

COMPROMISING

It is unlikely that you will find a perfect health plan with no compromise required. That should take some pressure off consumers worried they haven't found the perfect plan. There probably isn't one, and conversely there may be multiple reasonable options.

Ralph described figuring out there was no single ideal option available to him. "I had to compromise based on what was available. You've got to compromise both in terms of the health benefits, [and] in terms of the health costs. But in the end, I just took a look at it and said, 'Okay, do I really care as much about A, B, and C?' You alter your feelings a little bit if you've only got minimal selection. You can go with A or B. Well, you don't like A or B but, which is the lesser of the evils in your mind? And that's how you select."

Dave agreed that it is hard to get everything you might want or to even know what you might be trading off. "It's difficult to do that—I'm talking about just a cost comparison—and have a good sense that there won't be other charges thrown in." Even if you can anticipate hidden costs, he said, "That's just cost. Then there's level of quality. And so doing that kind of comparison, I could see optimizing for cost or quality, but not both." His solution is to find doctors whose judgments he trusts and "find the best ones I can access and take their recommendation."

Insurance decisions are complex, with seemingly infinite potential outcomes depending on where you go for care, what they charge, and what your health plan will cover. Acknowledge and accept that although options are not literally infinite, it can be difficult to accurately predict your future needs and optimize for them. By the nature of health insurance design, choosing the best plan for you will likely involve trade-offs between these factors. If you're not sure what services you'll need, try a few scenarios. Think about the worst case and the best case, and calculate how you'd fare financially in each one.

THE INDUSTRY COULD HELP

Industry participants like health plans and insurance marketplaces could adopt strategies and approaches to ease consumer challenges in choosing health insurance. "I think it's possible to simplify designs," Professor Newhouse suggested. "You [have] the various dimensions of the network. How broad the network is a good trade-off against the premium."

Curators of health insurance options could also limit people's opportunity to make selection mistakes by offering only high-value plans. "There is a role for the employer here," Newhouse continued. "And there's a role in the exchanges or marketplaces to limit the number of choices and the amount of variation that people have to contend with." Though employers already limit the number of choices they typically offer to a reasonably small number, they could focus on ensuring that high-value options dominate.

Newhouse conceded that curtailing choice won't work for all consumers. "There's obviously a trade-off there because you'll deny some people the choice they would like to have had." Still, he suggested the trade-off would be worthwhile for most people. "If you limit choice in a sensible way and help people, give them decision aids, that will all help the consumer."

Because some health plan components are standardized on the health insurance marketplaces, the agencies administering the marketplaces could make it clear to consumers which price components are set and which are variable across plans. "If you could somehow advise members of what was standard across different plans and what was a variable cost such that they could look to see which insurance carriers charge more for the variable cost, I think that'll help." McDevitt's example was on the Massachusetts marketplace; silver-level plans were required to have a $150 copayment on emergency room visits. "If you're a consumer, you don't know what's standard and what's not standard." If the agencies highlighted the variable elements, consumers could focus on those. Administrators could also develop a value score that combined all the factors and compared the relative value in an easy way for consumers to understand.

Making health insurance purchasing a truly consumer-grade experience is vital to improving the effectiveness of the consumer health insurance market. A consumer-grade health insurance process would involve clear, easy-to-use tools to compare health plan options on the bases that matter to consumers. Consumers also need to be able to see realistic scenarios so they can figure out the greatest-value plan for them. Such models need to allow for individual priorities and preferences, which may not be all about numbers. As Kayak and others like it brought airline ticket comparison and purchasing online, Hipmunk added an agony filter to help travelers understand the trade-offs they might make for a lower fare. So, too, should the state and federal marketplaces: move beyond simply putting health insurance purchasing online. Though that is a huge improvement over the old, manual comparisons people had to do, there remain opportunities to improve the experience for consumers. Many marketplaces are already making significant improvements. They should look to the best digital models and press on. And consumers should demand that they do.

13

Money-Back Guarantee

How to get what you pay for

"Having four kids means you're likely going to be using your health insurance, maybe more than other people," Angela explained her family's decision to choose a gold-level health plan—one of the most generous and costliest tiers under the Affordable Care Act—from among their options. From regular specialist visits for one daughter's Tourette's syndrome and another's migraines to her own talk therapy, someone in Angela's family always seemed to need something. One daughter fell down the stairs and appeared to have broken a toe. Another child needed a throat culture to rule out strep. Angela, herself, fell while chaperoning a school field trip and injured her knee.

This family might not quite qualify as what health plans call "high utilizers"—those members who use disproportionately more services, typically due to severe, chronic illness or catastrophic accidents, such as a transplant or recurring hospitalizations. But this middle-class family—living on the modest income from Angela's husband's university job and her own part-time nonprofit work—did use a lot of services. The encounters were leaving them financially vulnerable.

Over the past 15 years, the value of their health benefits had steadily eroded. When Angela's husband first started working at the university, his compensation included an allotment for the couple's health insurance. When their options began to include deductibles, the university would

189

pick up part of the cost—first $2,000, and then $1,000, of a $3,000 deductible. Like other employers fighting health care inflation, the university kept switching insurance carriers, taking advantage of insurers' willingness to cut deals to win their business. For a while, the university passed at least some of those savings onto employees.

When the ACA was enacted, Angela felt their options changed substantially. "They switched over and suddenly my husband got this tiny little bump in salary, and he started to have to pay the premium."

The family's financial strain compounded as they used more services. Angela's knee, injured on the school trip, got worse during physical therapy. Her doctor recommended an MRI, which the insurance company wouldn't approve until she had had an X-ray, which she knew would not show anything. "Everyone knew that it was a soft tissue issue," she said. "But I still had to get the X-ray and I still had to pay the copay to get the X-ray, and I still had to pay the charges that weren't being covered for the X-ray before they let me get an MRI."

As Angela was navigating her knee problem, her second daughter started having strange headaches. One night, the daughter lost her balance, fell against the wall, and tumbled down the stairs. "We were completely freaked out." With the help of their pediatrician, they jumped a four-month long wait to see a neurologist and got the MRIs needed "to rule out all the scary shit, which they did."

Then, Angela needed knee surgery, which she was still paying for two years later, using a payment plan she had arranged with the hospital to ease the cash crunch created by their out-of-pocket share. "I realized in the middle of all this, we had a surgery and five MRIs happen in our house and we didn't meet the deductible. We never got to a point where insurance was paying for anything."

The family's premiums were approaching $500 a month, and, with the out-of-pocket payments, Angela felt, "We were getting it from all sides." Taking time off work for medical and physical therapy appointments also ate into her work hours, and therefore, her income. At one point, Angela said to her husband, "If anything else happens and we have to add another balance on top of our balance, we're going to be paying for this till we die."

What value was Angela's family getting for its money, squeezed by rising health insurance costs?

CONSUMER-DRIVEN HEALTH INSURANCE GONE AWRY

Angela's experience illustrates how the rise of consumer-driven health insurance has increased financial burdens for consumers, even those with relatively good health benefits. As health care costs have risen overall, employers have increasingly shifted costs to their employees, who end up paying a bigger share of higher costs. As employees—and consumers more generally—shoulder a greater share of health care costs, the value of their insurance has eroded.

Ironically, consumer-driven health care was supposed to increase the value of health insurance. In her book *Who Killed Health Care*, Regina Herzlinger envisioned a system in which health insurers would offer a broader range of options to enable consumers to shop for and find their best-fitting plans. Drawing on consumer-grade information like that available in other consumer markets, savvy consumers would help move the market to deliver higher-value, more efficient health care services.

The goal of consumer-driven health care broadly was to enlist consumers in fighting rising costs, as they would search out and reward the highest-value plans, forcing costs down. Furthermore, by aligning financial incentives between consumers and payers, cost-sharing would suppress unnecessary utilization because consumers would think twice about over-using—and having to pay for—optional health services. High-deductible plans, then, were framed as mechanisms for enabling consumer power, allowing consumers to direct more of their health care choices.

In practice, consumer-driven health care has largely translated into shifting financial responsibility to consumers, via deductibles and other cost-sharing components. Employers and health plans embraced such insurance designs[1,2] as a way of mitigating rising costs.[3]

In other words, this narrow approach to consumer-driven health care succeeded in shifting costs but not in maximizing value. Studies show that cost-sharing depresses overall health spending[4,5] because consumers avoid not only unnecessary or unduly high-priced care,[6] but also necessary or preventive care,[7,8] including services that would be free by law under the ACA. Thus, cost-sharing does not turn people into savvy shoppers who judiciously avoid unnecessary care; it makes people avoid care altogether.

A 2019 study[9] showed that women who switched to high-deductible health plans delayed breast cancer screening and treatment, sometimes by many months. Surprisingly, the difference in delays between lower- and higher-income women was modest. That is, the suppressing impact of cost-sharing affected consumers across the income spectrum.

Another study[10] examined how high-deductible plans affect diabetes care. After transitioning to high-deductible plans, diabetic patients had fewer emergency department visits, fewer hospitalizations, and lower overall health costs, and their health outcomes on the whole seemed no worse. However, patients from low-income neighborhoods fared worse; they had significantly higher high-severity emergency room costs and more hospitalizations. While the study showed that everyone delayed care to some extent, cost-shifting exacerbated disparities among income groups in access to health care and health outcomes.

We should not be surprised by these recent findings. After all, the original intent of health insurance deductibles was to curtail service utilization. In the 1950s, in response to coverage limitations of the original Blue Cross health insurance scheme, private insurers created a new category of insurance—"major medical"—with more generous coverage limits. The catch: to get more coverage in the event of catastrophic expenses without paying a lot more in premiums, the insurers required policy holders to pay deductibles before insurance coverage kicked in. This design was intended to protect insurers from losses by preventing moral hazard, in which consumers only buy insurance when they know they need to use it. Deductibles were also aimed at reminding consumers that health insurance is a "purchasable product," not a free entitlement benefit, and to discourage "sniffle claims" for small-dollar, routine services that cost insurers a lot to process relative to their benefit. Major medical caught on in the decade following its introduction, covering more than 30 million people by 1961.[11] For nearly 70 years, insurers have deliberately used consumer cost-sharing to suppress health care utilization.

Joseph Newhouse designed and directed the famous Rand Health Insurance Experiment.[12,13,14,15] In that study, people who paid for a portion of their health costs used fewer services overall, without significant decreases in quality of care.[16] Newhouse confirmed that "cost-sharing tends to reduce both medically appropriate and medically inappropriate care . . . which suggested that suppressing the inappropriate care was actually suppressing some harms that offset, for most people anyway, the harms of forgoing the appropriate care." That is, avoiding care led people to avoid medical errors that can result in the course of seeking care. As Dr. Malaz Boustani bemoaned in Chapter 9, sometimes when people seek medical care, bad things can happen. Here, avoiding care prevented people from experiencing those bad things.

Despite these positive effects of cost-sharing, the impact was not equitably distributed, with lower-income people faring worse: the downsides of forgoing appropriate care tended to outweigh protection against bad care for lower-income people. "That finding, along with common sense, gave rise to a move toward making cost-sharing less blunt," Newhouse noted.

But cost-sharing has become anything but less blunt in recent years. Despite failures and unintended consequences of consumer-driven health plan designs, the trend persists. As discussed in Chapter 10, 82%[17] of employees now have deductibles, up from 63% a decade ago.

Not only are more people subject to deductibles, they are subject to higher deductibles. The average deductible nationwide is now as high as $1,800,[18] more than double the 2008 average.[19] Of those with deductibles, the majority had deductibles of $1,000 or more.[20]

Deductibles are not the only cost-sharing component pinching consumers. In 2018, nearly two-thirds (63%) of workers with copayments for primary care visits had to pay more than $20 per visit; that was true for less than one-third (29%) of workers a decade before.[21]

In Chapter 11, I discussed the rise of coinsurance—the percentage of health costs consumers pay directly. In 2018, the average coinsurance for office visits was 18%.[22] Nearly 20% of workers also had coinsurance for hospital services, with about three-quarters of workers responsible for more than 10% coinsurance.[23]

Additionally, premiums themselves increased by 20% between 2013 and 2018, almost double the rate of wage increases.[24] The average premium contributions paid by employees in 2018 was close to $1,200 for individuals and more than $5,500 for family coverage, representing a 65% increase (for families) since 2008.[25]

Between premium contributions and out-of-pocket cost-sharing, employees spent nearly $8,000 in 2018, or more than one-third of the cost of their health insurance. Employee out-of-pocket spending has risen by 67% since 2008, compared to the overall costs, which increased by 56%.[26] The JP Morgan Chase Institute, which tracks out-of-pocket health spending, found that one in six families made an extraordinary medical payment in any given year, associated with 9% higher credit card debt the following year.[27]

"There's no doubt that there are financial effects," continued Newhouse. "People are bearing more risk, and people that have serious health events are having trouble financing them." He noted that people with chronic diseases may be particularly at risk: "If you get a serious diagnosis, you have a serious cardiac problem or cancer or stroke, you could be wiped out by a big deductible, particularly if you have to pay the big deductible year after year."

That last point is critical: people with chronic diseases or ongoing health problems must satisfy their deductibles each year, but, according to Newhouse, the effect of cost-sharing on utilization is a one-time impact. Any deterrent cost-sharing provides to over-utilization is only evident immediately following the change; there is no ongoing reduction in utilization. In the Rand study, Newhouse said, "Once I increased the deductible and use has fallen, then I've done it." After those initial savings, cost-sharing only increases the financial burden on consumers; costs do not keep going down. "Increasing deductibles [is] basically a way of shifting at least some of that increase in costs to people that are using medical care and are most likely sick. But it does so at the price of increasing the risks they bear in the financial consequences."

Although cost-shifting to consumers has no ongoing financial benefit in terms of savings, employers and health plans continue to ratchet up consumer financial responsibility year after year.

EROSION OF HEALTH INSURANCE VALUE

The increasing financial burden from consumer-driven insurance designs hits individual health insurance purchasers hard. Jared, a former health care executive in between jobs, questioned the value of health insurance he bought on his state's insurance marketplace. I had scheduled an interview to get his expert opinions, but during our conversation, his personal perspective emerged.

Jared had bought family coverage on his state's health insurance marketplace, paying $2,500 per month in premiums, with a $2,500 per-head deductible, coinsurance, and a limited provider network. He saw value in the ACA options for lower-income people who qualify for cost reductions through subsidies but saw himself in "the worst possible place you can be, because you're paying all in." With costs so high, it did not make much sense to buy insurance through an exchange.

Worse than the absolute cost was Jared's sense that he was not getting value. "The product that you get, regardless of whether your premium is the full premium or something subsidized, it's inferior to what it was four or five years ago. And it's getting worse over time."

Jared had analyzed marketplace product offerings between 2014 and 2018. "It was a significant change in terms of the exchange. If you went to a public exchange, what you could buy in 2014 (or) 2015 versus today is significantly different. And the premiums are significantly higher. You've got a much more limited network."

Based on this value erosion, plus Congress's effective nullification of the individual health insurance mandate,* Jared predicted the demise of the unsubsidized individual insurance market. He might be right. As fewer people choose to buy less attractive marketplace plans, those who do will likely need it the most—the most costly individuals. Insurers will charge more to cover those more expensive members, further eroding value and dissuading others from buying in. At some point in that vicious cycle—sometimes called a *death spiral*—insurers who can't make money in the marketplace or who find the financial risks too high will exit the market. Fewer participating insurance carriers reduces competition, which in turn invites inferior or more costly products to the market.

In support of Jared's theory that the individual mandate is vital to marketplace success, data from Massachusetts—which implemented similar health reform years before the Affordable Care Act—show that once the

---

* In December 2017, the U.S. Congress passed the Tax Cuts and Jobs Act, which set the tax penalty for not having health insurance to $0, effectively eliminating the individual mandate, beginning January 1, 2019.

individual mandate was fully implemented, enrollment grew by nearly 27% and premiums dropped 23%.[28]

Prospective estimates of declines in enrollment resulting from undoing the individual mandate ranged from 3[29] to as many as 13 million.[30] After the mandate was effectively gone, enrollments—which had already declined from the high-water mark of nearly 19 million in 2015 to 14.4 million in 2018—declined by another 650,000, a 5% decline in the first three months of 2019.[31]

Absent some intervention or change in course, continued erosion of health insurance value seems likely if not inevitable.

THE NEW VULNERABLE

Shifts in the insurance market have created a new group of underserved consumers: not the very poor and vulnerable but those who don't qualify for public subsidies, get no help from an employer, or are lower-earning on high-deductible employer plans. These consumers—caught between deeper need and greater privilege—find themselves economically vulnerable without any source of support.

The *Los Angeles Times* profiled a family of five, saddled with $15,000 of medical debt, struggling to chip away at bills that had accrued from the premature birth of their second child and an ER visit for their youngest.[32] This family's experience resembled Angela's, facing a level of financial vulnerability not typically associated with the American middle class. When one of Angela's four children fell, they did not rush to the emergency room for what they thought was a broken toe. It was 8:05 P.M., and Angela said to her husband, "We have a choice. We can wait and see how she's doing in the morning, or we can go cough up $200 at the emergency department." They decided to wait. "I'm not destitute, but I had to really think hard about that."

Jared felt buffered from extreme vulnerability but recognized the financial jeopardy health insurance designs put many people in. "I think it's wrong for a family to possibly face bankruptcy if you get into the hospital, or something bad happens, and all of a sudden you're out-of-network. Now, I'm one of the families [that's] okay, but there are a lot of people that are not. . . . They go to the hospital and they get a $50,000 bill, and the guy makes $40,000 a year."

Huge medical bills create true financial crises. In 2015, one million Americans faced medical bankruptcy,[33] and two-thirds of people facing bankruptcy cited direct medical bills or related lost income as the cause.[34] More than $1.5 billion has been raised in 250,000 GoFundMe campaigns for medical expenses, representing one-third of all the money raised on that platform.[35] Though insurance is designed to provide protection against economic catastrophe, it simply does not provide enough protection for many Americans.

As much burden as huge medical bills place on individuals and families, ultimately bills often go uncollected. Only 68% of patients fully paid off medical bills in 2016.[36] Providers raise rates to recoup uncollected funds, which in turn strains patients financially.

Art, whose story appears in Chapters 5 and 9, had his medical bill forgiven, initially. He had switched insurance around the time he had surgery; when he gave the provider his new insurance information, the bill went up. "They had written me off as being a poor person. They wrote off 90% of the bill." This made no sense at all. "If I tell you I don't have insurance, I pay $500. If I tell you I do have insurance, I pay $750 plus the insurance company pays the rest of the bill? I'm incentivized to not have insurance." In theory, insurance should lower one's costs; when it doesn't, as in Art's case, it makes sense to ask, "Why bother?"

EXTRACTING VALUE FROM HEALTH INSURANCE

How can consumers get their money's worth in the face of declining value of health insurance, especially when insurance companies sometimes make it hard for consumers to use their benefits?

The story of Theo's colonoscopy in Chapter 5 showed how health plan rules can be a deterrent to using insurance at all. Rosemary found herself in a similar insurance maze. When her daughter was hovering at the bottom of the pediatric growth charts, Rosemary's husband joked, "She's really big for a two-year-old. But she's almost four!" Her daughter needed Prilosec to help her digestion, but it was non-preferred on the formulary and cost $50 per prescription. Preferred drugs that would have cost $20 weren't dosed for small children. Mail order would have been cheaper but wasn't an option because the drug needed to be refrigerated. With no preferred drug option for her daughter's age and size, Rosemary tried to get the health plan to authorize the non-preferred drug. "It's bullshit," Rosemary vented. "It's not my fault that she can't take one of the preferred drugs because she's only 27 pounds!" Rosemary appealed and even had the pediatrician advocate on their behalf, but the insurance company wouldn't budge.

For Valerie, the obstacle to capturing health insurance value was in how the rules were interpreted in the first place. A successful partner in a prestigious law firm, Valerie's family had met their $4,000 deductible. But she noticed they were still getting charged—$700 and counting—for services that should have been fully covered. When she called the health plan to resolve the discrepancy, a polite, well-meaning customer service representative—I'll call him Victor—said he would research the situation and call her back. He didn't. When Valerie called again, Victor told her the plan had zeroed out $800 of medical expenses incurred by one of Valerie's daughters who had recently turned 26 and started using COBRA to buy into her parents' plan. Backing out the $800 left the family under the deductible, even though they had already spent enough to satisfy it.

"Can you show me where in your plan documents is the language that you think allows you to do this?" Valerie asked Victor. A corporate attorney with expertise in class-action lawsuits, Valerie almost felt bad for him.

"Charges must be for a member," was roughly the language they read together on the health plan's website. "That doesn't really say you can do this," Valerie told him. Her daughter was a member when the expenses were incurred and still a member via COBRA. The costs were legitimate either way and should count toward the family's deductible—or her daughter's on COBRA—based on the health plan's own language.

He probably shouldn't have, but Victor agreed. "I have to say that is rather loose and vague language." Ever the lawyer, Valerie couldn't believe he would admit that on a recorded line and didn't want him to get in trouble. "So you don't get fired for saying that, let's hope I never have to use your admission," she said to him.

Fueled by a quest for fairness, amplified by concern for her daughter, Valerie didn't give up. She escalated through her company and eventually got the post-deductible charges reversed.

The health insurance bureaucracy was no match for Valerie, a uniquely qualified self-advocate. She read and understood her health plan documents, took the time to call and ask questions, and took steps to hold Victor—on behalf of the plan—accountable for a resolution. She recognized the plan's basis for zeroing out the charges as wholly inadequate to support their action. Valerie was also lucky to have a corporate sponsor behind her to amplify her message and seniority in her firm to get the internal attention that helped ensure a relatively rapid resolution. As the dispute worked its way through the process, she was able to float the money the health plan should have paid, where many people could not have.

While Valerie succeeded, she had several advantages that not all consumers have. As an educated, professional woman, she felt entitled to question the health plan and to push until she got adequate resolution, just as Austin had felt entitled to push for coverage of his asthma medicine, as described in Chapter 7. Valerie did not fear retaliation. She could afford to pursue resolution on principle, for fairness.

Still, she worried how others would fare in the same situation. "I can't be the only person who has had this happen," Valerie surmised. She is most certainly right; the problem was likely systemic, the resolution individual. That policy is probably built into the plan's systems or standard protocols, and possibly no one had recognized or challenged it before. Based on my professional experience, I could imagine the language had been written long ago and lived on through numerous generations of plan-rule documentation updates. In this type of convoluted bureaucratic maze, how vigilant must consumers be to extract value from their health insurance?

Health plans work hard to manage their financial risks. Among the strategies they employ—deliberate or otherwise—is bureaucracy. The hassle factor prevents consumers from fully capturing value to which they're entitled. This was Dave's interpretation of his health plan, anyway. "From the expense side," he said, "I'd probably need to spend half an hour every week just to stay on top of things for myself but also for the kids." He blamed the insurer's incentives; deterring consumers from capturing value is financially beneficial to the health plan. "Things are not laid out well to make it easy to get all that you're entitled to. The areas of full reimbursement and the areas where something was questioned have to be teased out by you looking at lots of paperwork online, and the reasons are buried in PDF documents. They're a couple levels down, using codes. It really creates some disincentives." Consumers have to overcome those barriers to even bother trying to capture value to which they're entitled.

Though Dave's insurance comes from a generous employer, he found it demeaning to have to work so hard to use his benefits. "If your credit card operated the same way and you had to go through each of your credits to find the mistakes and keep track of those and notify them, and if they were as complex as health care where you have partial coverage, formulas applied in different ways to different types of care, then the people would go nuts. But something about health care puts people in a position where they have to tolerate it."

Dave felt consumers have no choice, especially consumers who are handed preset choices by an employer. His coping mechanism is "to withdraw and not be as aggressive as probably would save me more dollars."

Is that what insurers and employers are counting on?

VALUE SEEKERS' SUCCESS

Sometimes, persistent consumers succeed in extracting, even maximizing, health insurance value. Doing so requires being undeterred by health insurance complexity, as well as careful advanced planning to take full advantage of benefits.

Phoebe, a young professional on leave from a high-paying corporate job to pursue a master's degree, described her quest for straighter teeth. "I've got Invisalign, specifically because the insurance is really good under my employer, so this will be the cheapest it probably will ever be for me." The main driver of her decision was a flexible spending account she figured she wasn't going to use otherwise, in which she had saved more than half the cost of Invisalign. Fear of losing the money she had responsibly put away for health expenses drove her decision making. Her employer—a huge global company—offered a robust dental plan and covered up to $2,500 of Invisalign costs. Phoebe shopped around and found that her dentist charged $3,500, better than an orthodontist who charged $5,000. With her company's contribution, she would basically spend just $1,000. To get that deal, she was willing to travel home—several states away—to see the dentist, with whom she had worked out a treatment plan to accommodate the distance. The savings made the inconvenience worth it to Pheobe.

Adam took value-seeking to a whole other level. A young father with a new baby on the way, Adam oversaw operations for a small company. Among his duties was choosing employee benefits. As the company was selecting their health plan for the coming year, Adam "did the math on it." A lower-deductible plan would save him so much money that it would be worthwhile to reimburse his colleagues for the premium difference between the higher- and lower-deductible plans. "Everybody else was single," he explained. "It was like the difference between $250 a month for them and $270 a month for them. They didn't want the lower deductible or the higher-coverage plan because they're a bunch of 27-year-old single people who are healthy. I really wanted it." He offered to pay each of his five colleagues the monthly difference in premiums, about $150 for several months. "We saved thousands of dollars having [a baby] on that lower-deductible plan."

That's value-seeking to a clever and somewhat extreme degree. Not everyone can save so much in this way, but there are ways average consumers can seek value.

HOW TO GET VALUE FROM HEALTH INSURANCE

Good value means getting your money's worth. Like many obstacles consumers face in getting value for their health care spending, the problem of eroding health insurance value is a hard one for individuals to fix. Voting with your wallet is not an option for many. More than half of Americans get their health insurance through their employers, who curate and narrow the choices. Among non-elderly adults, more than 27 million remain uninsured.[37] For people who buy individual insurance, choices may be narrowing; 17% had only one plan option in 2019, up from only 2% in 2016.[38]

Absent real flexibility and abundant consumer choice in health insurance of the sort envisioned by Regina Herzlinger, there are still a few ways to capture as much health insurance value as possible.

1. Read your plan documents

Painful as it is, it's vital to know your rights and your benefits. Those plan documents are considered a legally binding contract between you and the health plan.[39] Valerie's story is a powerful tale of reading—and questioning—the legalese on which the health plan operates. Few consumers have Valerie's level of legal expertise to challenge a flawed decision, but reviewing and questioning are still good practices. Timing and technicalities matter a lot in health insurance, so pay attention to the calendar and the details of procedures for appealing decisions, exceptions to coverage, and other specifics.

2. Don't trust; verify

Those plan documents are written in their own language and subject to wildly different interpretations. No matter how closely you read them, I hate to say it, but don't assume your interpretation is correct. Before you get health care services, call your insurance company and confirm that you know what is covered. Though you cannot prepare for extreme emergency situations, many care decisions allow time to clarify coverage.

Tara, a nurse and new mother, followed this strategy; even though she is well-versed in health care, she is not always certain of what services are subject to the deductible or what things will cost. "Every time I solicit any sort of care, I log into the website and see if it's covered, and find a provider, and then call them and make sure that they are covered."

I'd add from the wisdom of Valerie: Ask the health plan's customer service where in the plan documents the policy is referenced. Make sure it says what they claim it does.

3. Advocate and escalate

If you've read your plan documents, confirmed something should be covered, and still get a medical bill or insurance denial, argue it. You don't have to be a lawyer like Valerie to know when something doesn't seem right. Sometimes, a reasonableness standard applies to the enforcement of such rules, so your interpretation is highly relevant.

If you don't get a satisfactory resolution, ask to speak to a supervisor, manager, director, or vice president. If you can email or submit a request for resolution online, that gives you a paper trail to refer to if necessary. You might even try asking for the compliance department or for their legal basis for their decision. In *An American Sickness*,[40] Dr. Elisabeth Rosenthal provides templates for escalating about erroneous medical bills; the concepts can be adapted to advocating with health plans as well. Additionally, consumer advocates in nonprofit and government agencies may be able to help. You may not win in a fight with your health plan, and it may not feel worth the effort, but your willingness to escalate and pursue fairness and common sense will help get these issues on the leadership's radar. The best-quality health plans will take their members' concerns seriously.

4. Amplify

If you're on social media, use your voice if something goes wrong or you wind up in a protracted fight. Just be careful to stay within the boundaries of libel laws and basic civility. At worst, others with similar experiences will throw you some moral support. At best, a social media staffer, usually in the marketing department, will notice and escalate internally. No corporation loves public embarrassment, and marketing and communications staff are often the most attuned to the potential power of unhappy customers and may help put you on a path to resolution. It can't hurt to try getting attention through public means.

PART THREE

Getting Better

14

Everyone Has Teeth

Why dental care and coverage are separate from everything else and why that needs to change

---

"Why is it a privilege to get your teeth cleaned?" Bella asked. Just out of college, she was learning to navigate health insurance on her own for the first time. She opted not to buy dental coverage because the $100 extra per month did not seem worth it, especially on her recent-graduate wages.

"I wouldn't want to pay an additional monthly fee just to have it," she explained. "If I decided once a year I wanted to go to the dentist, I would just pay out of pocket." She assumed it might cost $75 or $100 for a cleaning. If so, it would make no sense to pay 12 times that in a year.

"I feel like it should all just be covered together." With the baggage-free eyes of a typical Millennial, she questioned why dental care isn't included with medical coverage. "What percentage of the population wears glasses or contacts? And is it the same number of people who need a gynecologist? If so, why isn't it covered?" Insurance covers lots of services that not everyone needs. Why aren't dental services included?

After all, as Bella noted, "We all have teeth."

IT'S NOT THE SAME

Even though we all have teeth, we don't all treat them the way we do the rest of our body parts. For many consumers, dental decisions are less serious than other health care decisions.

"Honestly, I chose a dentist based on proximity to my office and that was in my network," Emily, a Manhattan-based professional told me. When she had looked online for a dentist, she also checked patient feedback. "It was a really simple process." She assumed her dental care would focus on maintenance. "My teeth have never been a medical focus for me. I know I need to do it but I'm not willing to agonize over the decision." With cleanings three times a year and an occasional cavity filling, her experience has so far met her expectations. Her dentist's office is not the nicest, and she sees whichever dentist is on duty. And it's good enough. "I'm checking the box. I'm getting my teeth cleaned. I don't give a ton of thought to it."

By contrast, she painstakingly reviewed five different health plan options, extensively comparing the costs of fertility procedures she planned to undergo in the coming year. But for dental coverage, "I just picked the lowest."

Sophie, a self-described hypochondriac, also weighted medical and dental decisions differently. "Whenever I need a [medical] test, I just get it done right away because I'm so nervous about the outcome, I feel like I don't have the mental state to comparison-shop." She is more relaxed about dentistry. "I feel like with health care, at any moment there could be a life-or-death situation, even when you're going for a routine blood test. It just makes me really nervous." Yet her teeth don't worry her. "The worst thing that could happen with dentistry is you could have a tooth fall out or something like that. The stakes aren't as high."

THE ROOTS OF SEPARATION

The disembodiment of our teeth results, in part, from the different paths along which dentistry and medicine evolved.

In Steven Sondheim's musical *Sweeney Todd*, the title character—a murderous barber—wins a bet that he can outperform his rival in two services: a close shave and a tooth extraction.

In the 1800s, the care of teeth was entrusted to barbers like the fictional Sweeney Todd. Unregulated and trained only through apprenticeships, if at all, barber surgeons would roam, setting up shop temporarily to pull teeth, fill cavities, and sometimes transplant teeth from living or dead donors. Mary Otto's *Teeth*[1] details the horrors that could result from care by unskilled or unlucky practitioners. Dental procedures during this period often resulted in infection, in death, and in one unlucky patient part of a jaw coming off with several teeth still attached. Perhaps not surprisingly, Otto writes, "few maladies were viewed with more dread than diseases of the teeth."[2]

In the 1830s, two pioneers teamed up to professionalize dentistry. Chapin Harris, a dentist and avid student of dental phenomena, and Horace Hayden, an intellectual with varied scientific interests, sought to raise the level of knowledge and training in—and respect for—the dental profession. They founded a journal and professional society and tried to create a dentistry department within the University of Maryland's College of Medicine. The physicians in charge rejected their request, reportedly dismissing dentistry as having "little consequence."[3] Undeterred, the pair raised funds, petitioned the state legislature for a charter to establish a dental school, and opened the Baltimore College of Dental Surgery in 1840.

"From this very well-intentioned attempt to legitimize dentistry and provide better care for people came the separation that continued to spin out and become more and more and more distinctive," explained Lisa Simon, DMD, a dentist and fellow in oral health and medicine integration at the Harvard School of Dental Medicine (HSDM), who has written about the historical separation of dentistry and medicine.[4]

This original separation was further compounded as medical insurance evolved. As described in Chapter 10, American health insurance emerged in the 1920s as protection against catastrophic health events and associated expenses. Insured members paid regular small amounts into a pool intended to offset infrequent, large expenditures. Having paid into the shared pool, participants would get assistance covering extraordinary expenses if needed.

Conversely, dental insurance was designed to create incentives for steelworkers to pay union dues in the 1940s. Simon described the pitch this way: "Let me offer you this perk. What if we gave you discounted dental care for you and your kids and your wife?"

In the 1960s, when Medicare and Medicaid were established to provide health insurance for older and lower-income Americans, respectively, the American Dental Association successfully fought the inclusion of dental services, leaving the financing of dental care outside these safety-net insurance schemes from the start.

The American Medical Association also strenuously fought Medicare and Medicaid, fearing lower reimbursements and loss of control to government overseers. "The only real difference there is that the AMA lost and the ADA won," Simon noted. "But it's not like the dentists were more out for their own best interests than the doctors were. They were just better at it."

To this day, Medicare does not cover dental treatment, and Medicaid lets states decide whether or not to cover adult dental care; many do not.

Private dental plans are often sold and purchased separately from core medical plans, both in employer settings and on individual health insurance marketplaces.

"We're continuing to fund and pay for and think about [medical and dental coverage] separately," Simon said. "One is a necessity in the event of catastrophe and one is a perk."

AN ARMY OF ONE

Simon knows all too well the harm caused by the separation between oral care and medicine.

After practicing as a dentist, Simon enrolled in Harvard Medical School (HMS) with the goal of improving oral health through training and credentials from both sides of the divide.

In dental practice, she was "fundamentally heartbroken every day at being a clinician in that broken system." She had understood intellectually the impact of medical-oral separation, but living it made her feel "totally powerless to give people the care they needed." For high-blood pressure patients, she could not get a nurse from within the same clinic—just a floor below—to consult. She couldn't get social workers to call her back about patients with relapsed substance use disorder. If she prescribed antibiotics, there was no way to convey that to the primary care doctors. She simply did not fit into these clinicians' standard work flow.

Ironically, though Simon took her first-year dental school courses with medical students, she had to repeat that year when she enrolled in medical school. She also had to resign her HSDM faculty position because she was not allowed to be both a student and a faculty member simultaneously. "The dental school is not enough a part of the medical school for the time in medical school to have counted, but it is too much a part of the medical school for me to keep my faculty title. It's a good encapsulation of the disjunction." The system is not set up for what Simon was doing.

From her unique perch, she knows "exactly how little dentistry we get taught." Once, during medical training, Simon saw a patient with what she called "a very obvious oral health problem that no one had identified." She could make the diagnosis because of her dental training, but most medical professionals—let alone students—could not have. How many missed diagnoses occur because no dentist happens to be in the room?

Advanced head and neck cancer offers a stark example of the effect of inadequate attention to oral health. Of Medicare beneficiaries with these diagnoses, 90% had seen more than two doctors in the year before they were diagnosed, and 46% had seen 11 doctors or more.[5] Nearly *a dozen* doctors, on average, failed to examine patients' mouths, missing what would be obvious metastatic cancer.

Most hospitals are ill equipped to address dental needs, according to Simon.

> If you go to the emergency room with a toothache, they're going to look in your mouth. They won't be able to diagnose a problem with your tooth. They're just going to be like, "It looks like you have a bad tooth" and then they'll tell you to go to a dentist. There's no referral system, and 50%[6] of people who go to the emergency room for a toothache don't see a dentist in the six months after their emergency room visit and it isn't because their tooth got better. That's not how it works. Teeth don't get better until you see a dentist. They might get a prescription for an antibiotic and they might get a prescription for an opioid, but those are Band-Aids. They're not treatments. There's nothing these doctors can do.

Simon continued, explaining how structural barriers to integration hurt patients and create inefficiencies.

> When dental problems overflow into the medical system, they do so in ways that are costly, and unproductive and harmful for patients because the medical system has never accommodated caring for dental problems the same way they would, say, if you go to the emergency room with a dermatology problem or an ophthalmology problem. They're not going to be like, "We can't do anything for you." They won't say, "It's your eyes, we're not here for that." But if you go to the emergency room with a dental problem, that is exactly what will happen to you. There is no treatment apparatus for a dental problem within the [ER].

These gaps likely do not reflect malice, forgetfulness, or lack of time or interest but rather insufficient systems. Clinicians may want to help, but they are not trained to, nor are the mechanisms in place to support those intentions. In fact, doctors are trained *not* to order a test if they don't know what they would do with the results. "Looking in the mouth is ordering a test when you don't know what you're going to do with the result," Simon said.

MISALIGNED INCENTIVES

The history of separation between medicine and dentistry is compounded by diverging payment model trends that create incentives for different kinds of care delivery.

Medicine has been grappling with the endlessly escalating effect of fee-for-service payment schemes, in which doctors and hospitals are paid for each service they provide. To better align financial incentives between providers and payers, payments have shifted to per-head payments, or "value-based" reimbursement in which providers get paid set amounts per patient. Incentives move from providing the most care to providing the most appropriate care.

Conversely, dentistry is still almost entirely locked into traditional fee-for-service payments; the more services dentists perform, the more they get paid. "I don't think it's that dentists are more selfish," Simon told me. "It's that their incentives are very different. The average primary care doctor isn't making more money if they run more tests for you, but your primary dentist very well might."

Fee-for-service reimbursement may not directly lead dentists to perform more services than patients need, but it certainly rewards them financially for doing do. "If you're my patient, I make more money if your tooth is so decayed that you need a crown," said Simon. "As a patient, your best incentive is that you never get a cavity at all and your tooth stays perfect. I can probably help you do that. But that's not the way the financial incentives are. You're expecting [dentists] to provide care in their patient's best interest while putting them in a system that is in opposition to that."

Consumers are therefore left to wonder what influence financial incentives have on their dentists. Like bringing your car to a mechanic, the expert evaluating the problem benefits from finding the costliest solution.

Unfortunately, Simon acknowledged, "We have done a bad job in dentistry of aligning our incentives with the patient's incentives."

CASH AND CARRY

One consequence of dentistry's separation from medicine has been the exclusion of dental services from health insurance, which contributes to the uneven distribution of dental care and significant financial burdens for consumers.

While approximately 85% of non-elderly American adults[7] have medical coverage, dental insurance lags far behind. One-third of non-elderly American adults, and more than 60% of seniors, have no dental insurance.[8] Forty percent of dental spending is out of pocket, compared with 11% for health care overall.[9] Non-elderly adults also report greater financial barriers to dental care than to other medical care.[10]

Though low-income children typically get dental coverage via Medicaid, dental benefits for low-income adults are optional for states to offer. Only 28 states[11] cover nonemergency dental care for low-income adults on Medicaid and states sometimes scale back coverage when budgets get tight. Least able to absorb out-of-pocket dental costs, many low-income adults only access care when their oral needs become medical emergencies. As one Medicaid member said in a focus group early in my tenure leading the health plan's marketing efforts, "Medicaid will pay to pull my teeth, but they won't pay to clean them."

Dr. Brian Swann, chief of oral health at the Cambridge Health Alliance and assistant professor at the Harvard School of Dental Medicine, explained the predicament for low-income patients. "It's either emergencies, which means going to a hospital with a medical doctor who doesn't know much about oral health, who's going to give you two prescriptions, one for pain and one for the antibiotics. Sometimes patients who don't have the money may only buy the pain meds because that's driving you into that hospital. As a result, the patient is going to eventually return to the hospital in three or four weeks asking for more medications, which they're going to give you." In communities with no access to dental care, he continued, "you see increased opioid usage to deal with the pain; you will see obesity, and you see edentulism [the condition of toothlessness]. People have no teeth."

Though it varies by market, most dentists do not accept Medicaid because the reimbursement is so low compared to that in the private market, and balance billing—charging patients the difference between Medicaid reimbursement and customary dental charges—is prohibited. Low compensation from public-sector coverage leads to insufficient supply of dentists to care for low-income people. Therefore, even those with Medicaid coverage often have nowhere to go for care. Much of the industry is private, Swann explained, estimating that more than 100 million adult Americans are left out, with no oral health benefits.[12]

"[It's] all about the money," Swann said bluntly. Dentists graduate with $300,000 to $400,000, or more, in debt, and many feel that the only way out of that level of debt is to join the private sector. "The public gets left out."

A huge swath of consumers is underserved, without dental coverage or the funds to pay out-of-pocket fees. Some dental chains do target lower-income consumers, but most providers ignore those consumers. The market, therefore, seems ripe for new approaches to distribute lower-cost dental care to a broader assortment of consumers.

In the meantime, the gap in the market creates gross inequities. "Oral health is a marker of inequality in America," said Dr. Shenam Ticku, instructor at the HSDM. "If you have the economic means, you can access care, which is not the same for most health [care]." Oral disease impairs quality of life through pain, social stigma, and lost productivity. "You don't think of that unless you have it," Ticku said.

Simon analogized the access problems posed by separation of dentistry and medicine as "walking through two sets of doors instead of one. If you don't have problems walking through doors, that probably isn't a big deal to you. . . . It is not an enormous burden to you to pay out of pocket for a filling, to remember to call your dentist every six months." People like this "are also unlikely to ever have a toothache in their lives. . . . But the people who have trouble walking through doors are most likely to suffer horribly from not accessing that second set of doors." For vulnerable consumers, dentistry offers a "less patient-centered system."

UNCOVERED

Even people with dental coverage do not get much financial relief when they actually need care. Swann argued the average $1,000 annual dental benefit limit is insufficient given that "dentistry also is the highest percentage of out-of-pocket costs in health care."

As discussed in Chapter 10, Lauren told me how access to ACA health insurance enabled her to start her own firm by protecting her financially from catastrophic health expenses. On the other hand, she learned the hard way that dental coverage offered much less protection. "There's a limit to what they'll pay, and the rest is your responsibility. I pay $139 per month and the limit is $1,000."

When Lauren's son broke a tooth, the dental staff told her, "Your insurance hasn't kicked in yet. . . . You have to pay six months before you get the benefits."

"So I pay now and they reimburse me?" Lauren asked.

"No," they said. "You're not entitled to benefits."

That prompted Lauren to look harder at her coverage. Benefit caps on top of delayed coverage made it barely worth the price she had paid. "It's really more economical to pay out of pocket."

Amelia similarly learned through personal experience that dental benefits don't cover much. When she moved away for graduate school, she signed up for university health insurance but not dental. Before her generous employer coverage expired, she stocked up on any dental care she might need for the foreseeable future. During school, she traveled home for regular cleanings and made sure they never did anything extra. "I wasn't afraid to be vocal about that," she said, guarding her wallet.

After graduation, Amelia spent more than $2,000 out of pocket when a broken filling led to a root canal and then a crown. The dental insurance she had bought with her individual health insurance paid for none of it. "That shitty exchange insurance only covers cleanings," which hadn't been clear from the plan documents. "What is the point of paying $50 a month for dental insurance if it only covers $200 a year worth of cleaning," she wondered. "That was eye-opening. It was such a scam!"

Amelia looked on the bright side of a bleak dental experience. "At least, getting a root canal made me realize I don't need to pay for dental insurance anymore. I guess it saved me some money that way. But it didn't pay for the root canal."

Tessa also learned the limits of dental coverage. After getting a crown that her dentist admitted "didn't go as well as I would have liked," she still needed a root canal. After all that work, the distance between that tooth and its neighbor was too large. "I have to floss ten times a day." The dentist suggested he redo the crown. Though the space annoyed her endlessly, she didn't address it right away. Her mouth, and her psyche, needed a break. Tessa came back months later to find a new dentist had taken over. She told him the tale of the too-wide gap. "You should've had that redone right away," he lectured. Couldn't he redo it now? she wondered. "Your insurance won't cover it because it's been less than five years, so it would cost $1,400. But you should get this done. It's really going to be better for your gums." The faulty procedure had essentially used up her dental benefits for five years; the financial burden of fixing it fell to her.

Lauren, Amelia, and Tessa discovered what insiders know: dental insurance isn't really insurance. Whereas insurance is designed for high-dollar, low-probability events for which it is hard to plan, dental care is often preventive, routine, and relatively low cost; even higher-ticket dental services can often be planned.

True to its origins, dental coverage is less insurance and more a discount plan to encourage preventive care. "The worse the problem, the more of the bottom line you're on the hook for," Simon explained. "Which is the exact inverse of what medical insurance is."

Mislabeled and misunderstood, dental "insurance" is at best a generous employer's contribution to offsetting costly dental care. More often, though, it is a disappointment to consumers who think they have insurance coverage. When they realize coverage can cost more than it delivers, consumers often determine that they are better off without it, if they can pay out of pocket. As long as dental coverage fails to deliver real value, dental insurers are inviting consumers to work around them and leaving lower-income people with insufficient care. Along the way, these companies are missing opportunities to build compelling consumer products.

THE ART OF DENTISTRY

Not only can value in dental coverage be elusive, it can also be difficult for consumers to know what care they really need.

"Dentistry is still based on the clinician's perception of what you need as a treatment," said Dr. German Gallucci, DMD, PhD, chair of the restorative dentistry and biomaterials sciences at the HSDM and a practicing clinician who oversees the Harvard dental clinics. He explained, for an extensive cavity, three different dentists might use three different approaches, each one potentially justified. "There is a huge spectrum on when the intervention needs to happen and what type of intervention needs to happen."

Simon agreed. The range of appropriate treatments Gallucci described can confound consumers trying to figure out whom to trust. Different options might lead people to assume dentists are "blindly picking and choosing what they want to bill you for." But dentists can have legitimately different philosophies. Where Simon might recommend watching a small cavity in someone with good oral care habits, another dentist might see risk in waiting and suggest filling it, independent of any profit motive. It could be "because they really do have a different philosophy of treatment."

But after dental work has begun, decline can be inevitable. "Once you have a filling, the consumer needs to understand, that is the beginning of the death cycle of that tooth," Fay Donohue, a former dental plan CEO, explained. Most dental work simply won't last forever. "The filling will fall out and then instead of a two-service you need a four-service and then the four-service falls out and then you need a crown and then that falls off. And then you need root canal. Finally, you'll lose the tooth and you'll need a bridge. That's what happens. So, you want to keep a tooth healthy."

For his part, Gallucci practices with long-term sustainability in mind. "I like to solve problems with the least interventional approach at each step," he said. Teeth "are among the few tissues in the body that do not regenerate. Every time you take something out of the tooth with your drill or with your instruments, it doesn't grow back." He tries to prolong the life of the natural tooth, though recognizes it's not always possible. "If you have a small decay, or if you have a medium-size decay and you treat it with a direct composite and the patient [has] that composite for seven years to ten years, and then needs re-intervention, I consider that successful."

"You can still use the other two options that you've had in the beginning," Gallucci continued. "Now, if you do the most invasive option at the beginning, then 10 or 15 years down the road, maybe the whole tooth is compromised. And now the intervention is bigger." The dentist has no options at that point.

How common is Gallucci's approach? I asked him. "I call this 'the experienced approach,'" he said and laughed. Informed by research, practice, and teaching dental students, he believes "dentistry is best, or patients are best served, when you achieve the maximum outcome with the least amount of intervention."

The Atlantic published an article[13] about unfettered over-treatment which reported that patients did not necessarily trust the new dentist who took over when an aggressive dentist retired. Patients had been told for so long that procedures were necessary and were skeptical when the new dentist saw no need to intervene. Gallucci also had this experience; he did not think a patient who had had multiple interventions needed anything more. It must not have sounded right to the patient. "I never saw the patient back," he said. "At the end, it's the patient's call."

WHO DO YOU TRUST?

If dentistry is an art, then how should consumers evaluate dental quality? And what should consumers do if two wildly different opinions can both be valid?

"It's true with everything in health care," Fay Donohue said. "If you've got an answer for how I can judge whether or not my PCP is any good, great! I don't think we've got a good answer."

"It's tough," Lisa Simon said. "Because a lot of it is on gut feel." If you trust or connect with one dentist over another, Simon recommended, follow your instinct. You might even tell one dentist what the other one said. "A good dentist—the right dentist for you—will say, 'That's reasonable,'" and explain their thinking. Ultimately, Simon said, "if your spider sense is tingling, this is not great." Listen to that instinct, she advised. If something doesn't feel right, pay attention. But it is not necessarily problematic if different dentists use different approaches. A dentist giving a second opinion might well say, "I can see why they'd say you need a filling for this tooth, but I actually wouldn't treat it just yet."

Donohue also cautioned consumers not to judge quality solely on how much a dentist wants to do. "You may have had a conservative dentist who watched and waited, and that was his practice and it worked really well for you." She suggested asking questions; if you get any resistance to your questions, be careful. "A good practitioner will want to share the information, will want to give you his reasoning or her reasoning, will want you to be an engaged consumer." If you feel a dentist is urging you just to trust him or her, "Go back to trust, but verify." Donohue suggests saying, "I do trust you; I'd like to see the evidence."

THE CASE OF THE MISSING CODES

One reason it is so challenging to evaluate the quality of dental care is the lack of diagnostic codes. Bear with me; this explanation requires a brief detour into the weeds of billing codes.

In medicine, clinical services are coded by diagnosis and treatment, allowing analysis connecting the two. Simon told me the codes "are hilariously specific," including things like, "sucked into jet airplane," "jet engine first encounter," "sucked into jet engine second [encounter]." However comical, the level of detail allows analysis of the appropriateness and effectiveness of the treatment for a given diagnosis, however rare being sucked into a jet engine may be.

In dentistry, however, there are no uniformly applied diagnostic codes: just billing codes that capture the procedures a dentist performs but not why he or she performed them. Simon explained, "I can say I did a filling. I don't say you had a cavity and therefore I did a filling." It is impossible, then, to detect inappropriate over-treatment, except in the most extreme cases. "There are no checks and balances."

If diagnostic codes are necessary to set quality measures and standards—and there are none in current dental practice—on what basis are dentists operating today?

"There *are* dental quality standards," Simon assured me. "But they're limited because you can only base them on the information we have, which is that things were done and not why we did them." The available process measures do not definitively show whether people are getting high-quality—or the right amount of—care. Available data can mask both over- and under-treatment. "You need to have quality measures to make sure that not only are people getting cheap care or affordable care, but any care. It is the pull to the push of a capitated system."

The implication for consumers is that "it makes it harder for me to tell patients that they can trust their dentist. To enter [a health care relationship] worrying that someone's going to try and stiff them a couple hundred dollars or whatever the case may be, I think that that builds a fundamental tension within dental care that's not fair and that leads people to feel even more anxiety about something they already feel anxious about on average."

Concretely, it also frames benefit limitations. Because there's no way to tell if a procedure is truly necessary, dental insurers simply set limits to prevent unfettered over-treatment. But those limitations can also arbitrarily prevent people from getting care they genuinely need, as Tessa experienced when she needed to repair a faulty procedure.

Benefit limits as de facto treatment guidelines cut both ways. "Just because it's paid for does not mean that everybody needs it all," Donohue reasoned. Coverage is not the same as a treatment recommendation. Consumers should focus instead on what they specifically need. "Every mouth is different," Donohue said. If you've never had a filling, you may not need as much monitoring or intervention as someone with a mouthful of them.

WHAT MEDICINE CAN LEARN FROM DENTISTRY

Dentistry needs improvement in many areas—from the inequitable access to the high out-of-pocket costs, the lack of financial protection that real insurance could provide, and the absence of quality standards to help build consumer trust. The great chasm separating oral care from the rest of medicine makes no anatomical sense and misses opportunities to improve patient care and well-being.

Despite these challenges, American dentistry also offers some key lessons for the rest of medicine:

1. **Price transparency:** The last time I had my teeth cleaned, the hygienist went out of her way to tell me the cost of fluoride had gone up, from $11 to $37. I asked why and learned they had not raised the price in a decade, and they were now out of step with the market. This interaction underscored dentistry's primary advantage over medicine: costs are explicit. Consumer responsibility is clear, and there are few, if any, financial surprises in dentistry, the upside of having to pay for so much out of pocket. Because patients are paying, they must consent to the costs. Price transparency is such a strong norm in dentistry that Donohue suggested caution if a dentist won't tell you their prices. "That's not a good answer," because dentists' fees are no mystery.

2. **Dentists know their business:** Though many doctors claim ignorance over costs and insurance intricacies, dentists are often deeply informed and involved in the financial aspects of their business. A private-sector dentist I interviewed is a preferred dentist in ten different insurance plans. "You have to keep that all straight," she said. Another dentist recited intricate details of several plans. Dealing with insurance and billing every day, she said, they know exactly what things cost and what to expect for reimbursement.

3. **Help with navigation:** As transparent as dentistry can be regarding costs, dental benefits are still confusing. Dentists told me that patients rarely understand their coverage completely. Dentists, therefore, try to help patients decipher and actively manage benefits, sometimes by optimizing coverage across benefit years, like if a patient is approaching their benefit limit for the year and could get part of the treatment in the following year. Dentists often offer payment plans and interface with insurance companies on patients' behalf. Amelia stayed loyal to her dentist even after moving out of state in part because of the administrator, who efficiently helped Amelia get reimbursed for bills she paid out of pocket. "She is like my best friend and made getting dental care very easy." Unlike consumers who get stuck in medical provider-insurer disputes, as described in Chapter 7, dental offices often provide valuable help navigating reimbursement.

4. **Consumer control:** The revered economist Kenneth Arrow argued that health care is simply un-shoppable—too different from other markets, demand being unpredictable and supply unknowable to consumers.[14] But dentistry offers a viable counterpoint. Consumers often

decide what dental care they get and when. "You have the sector of the health care economy where consumers do pay at least half of all costs," Donohue said, though consumers don't always realize they can direct their care. "It is stunning how little people think about it. It is information that is readily available in terms of the cost because most dentists have a fee schedule. They will tell you. They have to, because you're going to pay part of it."

Dentists have technical expertise that warrants respect; they have power and influence while the patient is in their chair. But these professionals know who pays a substantial portion of their bill and recognize consumers' decision-making power. As the financial equation in medical care shifts more heavily toward consumer responsibility, consumer opportunities to shop—or exert financial power—will likely increase.

American dentistry is clearly a consumer service. Dentistry has more explicit room than most parts of medicine for consumers to shop and to have a say in their own care. For better and worse, consumers are on the hook financially, and in return have opportunities to help shape their care. Dental care can be a nightmare, but it can also be straightforward and transactional. The dentist has clear authority and expertise, yet everyone knows who ultimately pays the bill.

WHAT CONSUMERS CAN DO TO GET VALUE FROM THEIR DENTAL SPENDING

To navigate flaws in the U.S. dental system, there are ways consumers can increase the value they get.

1. Focus on prevention

"Proper attention to the cleanliness of these organs contributes more to their health and preservation than is generally supposed," noted Chapin Harris, one of the founders of American dentistry.[15] More than 100 years later, I heard this message consistently from dental experts. The best way to get value from your dental care is to make sure you need as little of it as possible.

"If you actually take care of your teeth, then you should reduce the incidence of higher-cost procedures," Fay Donohue explained. "Prevention does work."

German Gallucci also emphasized prevention. "Dental conditions, for the most part, are preventable, highly preventable." In Switzerland, where Gallucci trained, students get regular hygiene checks and access to fluoride. "And the incidence of dental caries [cavities] or periodontal disease is one of the lowest in the world."[16]

2.   Ask for the evidence

Donohue is not a dentist but advises everyone to ask their dentist for evidence. "I would just ask the questions that you would ask about your health. Do I need it? What is the alternative? And then, if there's anything that I was uncomfortable with for a minute, I would look at getting a second opinion." She suggests asking, "What is the evidence?" If you know your mouth, you can ask about your specific situation and what's appropriate for you.

Though clear evidence does not exist for all of dentistry, where there is evidence, consumers should arm themselves with it. "You have to dig," Donohue said. Cochrane[17] and the American Academy of Pediatric Dentists[18] publish guidelines. Though many point back to asking your dentist, they at least provide a starting point of what to ask.

3.   Negotiate—if not for money, then for treatment options

Before asking about money, ask if there might be a lower-intensity treatment option to try. Lisa Simon suggested that if your dentist says you need a crown, "You might be able to say, 'Could we try a filling first?' And a dentist I would trust would say, 'I really do think it's going to go to this point and you should be prepared for that, but I can try.'" That's not to say every tooth can get filled before needing a crown, but it's a valid request, and it might be worth the attempt.

Donohue suggested consumers ask, "Before we talk about money, let's talk about do you need it in the first place."

In dentistry, people sometimes get treatment in advance of a problem, in case one develops. The best example is wisdom tooth extraction. "We do millions of dollars' worth of asymptomatic wisdom teeth," Donohue said. Obviously, symptomatic, painful wisdom teeth need to come out. But if one of yours needs to come out, do they all need to? "If it's simply more convenient and might help you in the future, is there any other part of your body that you would remove when that's the answer? I might get appendicitis." But rarely do people undergo an appendectomy because it might cause a problem in the future. Use common sense, and be willing to ask the questions.

There are some parts of dentistry where it may be possible to negotiate on price, or at least to shop around, like in orthodontics—but people rarely do. "You've got all kinds of opportunities," Donohue said; there may be dramatic price differences between providers. "You have to be [a] very wise consumer. Paying attention, feeling comfortable and understanding . . . exactly what you want." It may be possible to work with your orthodontist to target your treatment plan to a more limited scope to save money, but even just comparing providers can sometimes yield savings. Phoebe, introduced in Chapter 4 and discussed in Chapter 13, found financial rewards by shopping around. In my own family, we visited a second orthodontist and saved more than $1,000 for the same service.

4.   Be wary of marketing

Simon suggested caution with dentists who offer discounts for cleanings and X-rays. "That implies they're really trying to hustle patients." Gallucci also bemoaned commercial interests in dentistry. "Unfortunately, dentistry has been heavily influenced by marketing. I said unfortunately because when you look at the marketing strategies, they are oriented to maximize patient flow, and to maximize profitability." By implication, the focus on prevention and clinical quality may lag behind profit motives.

A dentist in private practice suggested that consumers should look at how dentists present themselves to the public. Is their website professional? Do they seem overly promotional or "cheesy," which may indicate they are working too hard to drum up business? A great reputation should help them fill their schedule without much marketing, she said. Consider the dentist's education, time in practice, and practical factors like location and insurance participation, if applicable. Then, use the first visit to evaluate the dentist. This dentist told me that early in her private practice a few patients sought to interview her before committing to becoming patients. "That's just not an accepted practice" in dentistry, at least not in her market, the way it might be in some fields, she explained. That time is not compensated and "it's conveying a lack of trusting." But she knows new patients evaluate her during the first visit. During "the comprehensive exam," she said, "I feel like I'm on a job interview."

Another private-practice dentist told me she used to offer promotions or discounts as a new practitioner. Now that she is well established, her practice grows by word of mouth. She's so busy with loyal patients who give her positive reviews she has stopped participating in some insurance networks, which means, ironically, they reimburse her more. Even without insurance referrals, this dentist maintains her busy schedule because of her great reputation.

5.   Demand the future

This book is intended to help consumers navigate the health care system, not to tell the health system experts what to do to improve the system; they likely already know. But the status quo has a powerful grip and often prevents insiders from reforming their own system.

One way to break the hold of the status quo is for the public to demand change. Dentistry has so much potential to become more cost effective, deliver higher quality, and become more accessible to more people. Consumers can help bring about such a future by demanding the improvements experts envision. Here are some developments to ask for.

1. **Integrate dentistry and medicine:** Better integration between oral health and medicine would improve consumer convenience and patient safety. The current separation requires patients to remember—and share—their medication information. Simon said, "People have to be more advocates for themselves than would be ideal [and] that becomes even more burdensome the sicker you are or the lower health literacy you have, and those are the people who are most at risk for something bad happening to them as a result, and vice versa."

   For vulnerable populations and medically complex patients, more effectively linking dental and medical care maximizes the number of touchpoints with patients, which yields more opportunities for dentists to help identify and address care needs. Screening patients while they're in the dental chair is effective, if clinicians are trained and compensated for that, and if systems are in place for them to make the appropriate clinical connections on behalf of those patients. "There's no system set up to incentivize these kinds of things even though they would definitely benefit patients," Simon noted.

2. **Increase access to preventive dentistry:** Just as primary care providers have been transforming themselves into "medical homes" that centralize and offer a full spectrum of patient care, Gallucci suggested creating dental homes. Longstanding, trusting patient-dentist relationships could focus on prevention and help patients who require extensive intervention navigate more complex care and oversee treatment plans. "Dentists are not doing that," Gallucci lamented. "They're just doing intervention. A broken tooth, we fix it, and then we move on. We need to reinforce that notion that dentists are in essence health care providers and they should be watching for the oral health of the patient." Today, dentists typically focus on treating problems instead of on monitoring and maintaining oral health. "Somebody would have to pay for that because I don't think that there's enough [revenue in preventive care] to maintain a facility under those conditions," Gallucci said. But such a philosophical and practical shift could "essentially change the course of dentistry."

3. **Break the office walls:** "Dentistry for centuries has been a tailor-made discipline," Gallucci offered an analogy. "Before industrialization of clothing, the only way to have a nice suit or a nice dress was to go to a tailor. Then you have all these machines that sew and made it faster,

with standard sizes. Now you can buy a suit for less than hundred dollars. Dentistry is entering that phase now with digital dentistry," which, if used as a public health tool, could improve access to care.

Gallucci noted three levels of barriers to oral care: (1) financial limitations or lack of affordability, (2) insufficient supply of dentists in a particular geography, and (3) lack of qualified dentists in a particular area. Most people focus on the financial aspects of accessibility and appropriately so. But an unevenly distributed supply of dentists creates barriers as well. At the end of 2018, there were nearly 6,000 dental care Health Professional Shortage Areas (HPSAs) and almost 60 million people living in such areas.[19]

Shortages can impact care when, for example, a patient needs a crown but only has access to a dentist who does not do crowns. That patient may wind up with an unnecessary extraction. Digital dentistry would allow a properly trained clinician to scan the patient's mouth, fabricate a crown, and use a small machine to mill the crown essentially on the spot for a low cost. This type of 3D printing is already happening in fee-for-service dentistry. The technology is already here. "It's just never been thought of as a public health tool," Gallucci said.

Thus, the opportunity exists to "[take] away the tailored approach to dentistry, by putting more in an industrialized way leading to a cost reduction in delivery of dentistry."

An extension of digital dentistry is teledentistry, in which scans can be sent remotely to specialty providers. Then, it is only a matter of time before this technology gets attached to a smartphone, allowing consumers to scan themselves and automatically identify decay or disease. These technologies exist today and could be deployed to solve challenges of access, affordability, and trust in dentistry, according to Gallucci. "Now, the patient doesn't rely on what the dentist says but the patient sees it."

LEARNING FROM EACH OTHER

The historical separation between medicine and dentistry has consequences for the way Americans access care and contributes to suboptimal outcomes in both medicine and dentistry. Financial interests keep this separation firmly entrenched. Access is uneven. And costs come disproportionately out of consumers' pockets.

Everyone should have access to oral care. We should care about oral health in its own right, not just because good oral care might also contribute to improving medical outcomes and lowering health care costs. As Lisa Simon said, "Fundamentally, not having pain your mouth and having this part of your body remain whole and healthy is important on its own."

Still, dentistry has lessons for the rest of medicine about consumer roles. Consumers clearly pay for their dental care and are treated like customers as a result. Even though consumers—and physicians—have often been trained to take dental care less seriously than medical care, there are opportunities for medicine to look a little more like dentistry in terms of price transparency, patient involvement in clinical decisions, and greater consumer assistance in navigating the health care system.

15

Keep Your Government Hands off My Medicare!

What everyone else can learn from savvy seniors

"I never really thought of switching," Bernice told me about her health plan. A retired nurse-turned-family-therapist, Bernice was three weeks from her 88th birthday when we spoke about her experience with Medicare. "There's open season every year, but it works, and what's the point?" Bernice had retired as the clinical director of a mental health center and was more than capable of navigating her health insurance options. She simply felt no need to shop around.

I rarely meet people who are truly satisfied with their health insurance. Bernice seemed like an exception. Despite "a huge variety" of Medicare plans, her choice is simple. "The coverage is good. There's a wide network of physicians." While out of state a few years prior, she had sought care at an urgent care center. "They covered that. No paperwork. It was wonderful."

"Simple" and "wonderful" are not words often associated with health insurance in America.

While virtually all Americans age 65 and over are eligible for Medicare, many buy supplemental plans, too. Bernice's supplemental plan offered overseas coverage, which suited her aspirational travel bug. As Bernice increasingly struggled with mobility, her dream of exploring the world—especially Iceland—was fading, as was the value of travel benefits. Still, she stuck with her health plan.

Helen, another retiree, also stuck with her Medicare supplemental plan but was willing to consider other options. "It's good to look at it," she opined. When we met in her senior-living apartment, her white hair was cropped in a contemporarily stylish bob cut. She wore a perfectly flattering shade of deep magenta lipstick; her thick-black-rimmed glasses made her look like she belonged in a TV ad for some store or product trying to convey, perhaps, that "90 is the new 60!" The afternoon light softened as we spoke, highlighting her beauty. Born in the "socialist part" of Brooklyn to immigrants from eastern Europe, Helen's first language was Yiddish. She had taught in a large community college until she was 87, officially retiring at age 75 but staying part-time because she "just needed to be with people."

It did not surprise me that this 92-year-old widow would take the time to review her health plan options each year. Her small apartment was lovingly decorated with the signature eclecticism of someone who has collected a lifetime of treasures. The surfaces of various side tables were piled with orderly stacks of books and papers and envelopes, into which she dug at one point for a specific piece of mail she knew held the precise answer to one of my questions.

With no children, Helen independently handles her administrative life. "I'm my own manager," she said, in contrast to friends who refer such matters to their adult children. She balances her checkbook every month to test not only her finances, but also her mental acuity. She can usually "get it down to the penny," though she allows herself a ten-cent mistake. If she can't do it anymore, she'll know "I've lost it."

Despite her keen attention to details, and her annual review of her options, Helen does not see the benefit of switching health plans. "I don't see that much difference and I'm just comfortable with it." I might call this informed inertia. Whatever forces are at work, Helen's unwillingness to switch signals that something about it works for her.

As I interviewed more consumers over 65—a dozen in total—I started to realize they resembled savvy health care shoppers. Might older consumers hold the key to making consumer health care markets work for more Americans?

MEDICARE: THE BASICS

The health care system for older Americans is structurally different than for most others, and it enables a level of shopping, consumer choice and empowerment, and financial protection sorely lacking elsewhere in American health care.

Medicare is best known as the federal government health insurance available to most Americans 65 and older and some younger people with disabilities, who represent 15% of beneficiaries. The program was created in 1965 and signed into law by Lyndon B. Johnson after previous failed attempts to create universal health insurance under Presidents Truman and Kennedy.[1]

Over time, adjustments to the program expanded eligibility to cover non-elderly, high-need populations and to plug other coverage holes, resulting in a patchwork. For example, in 1980, President Carter signed a law allowing Medigap (or supplemental) plans and bringing such plans under federal oversight. In 2003, President George W. Bush signed into law Medicare Part D, which took effect in 2006, after previous attempts to create prescription benefits had been passed and repealed.[2] The 2003 law also renamed a prior program—Medicare+Choice—to Medicare Advantage, the comprehensive managed care program we have today. These changes have transformed Medicare from a basic safety net into a broader set of health insurance programs.

Today, Medicare comprises 15% of the U.S. federal budget, on par with total annual defense spending. In 2017, there were $702 billion in total Medicare expenditures, approximately $300 billion each on hospital and outpatient services and $100 billion on pharmaceuticals.[3] Medicare expenses almost doubled in the ten years from 2007 to 2017 and are projected to double again by 2027.[4]

Medicare is a bit of a beast in size and scope and a little like Frankenstein with an array of parts stitched together to make a whole program. And it's working for a lot of people.

THE BUSINESS OF MEDICARE

In modern political debates over expanding Medicare to cover more Americans—so-called Medicare for All—many people think of Medicare as the epitome of one-size-fits-all, socialized medicine, the opposite of a market-based approach.

It's not.

Far from a pure government health care program, Medicare has become a hybrid of public and private coverage, with attributes of both market force and regulation. Funding is similarly blended from a mix of beneficiaries' own payroll deductions during their working years, premiums current beneficiaries pay, and general revenues, as in, taxes.[5]

Along with core coverage, most of the 60 million Medicare beneficiaries also enroll in private health plans.[6] Approximately one-third (34%) enroll in Medicare Advantage plans; enrollment is even higher in some states, like Minnesota, where more than half[7] of Medicare beneficiaries enrolled in Medicare Advantage in 2018.

Medicare Advantage plans offer comprehensive coverage, limit enrollees' out-of-pocket liabilities, and cover extra benefits not offered under core Medicare. The average monthly Medicare Advantage premium in 2019 was $29 across all enrollees—or $65 per month for enrollees who pay premiums at all,[8] costs which have been steadily declining—yes, *declining*—since 2015.[9]

While some people assume Medicare Advantage is for wealthier people, it actually appeals to a diverse population. Compared with traditional Medicare, slightly more women enroll (57% vs. 53%), as do racial and ethnic minorities (29% vs. 21%) and lower-income people. In fact, 29% of Medicare Advantage enrollees earn $50,000 per year or more compared with 38% on traditional Medicare.[10]

Like HMOs, Medicare Advantage plans offer enrollees a sort of one-stop shop for the disparate parts of Medicare coverage. This cohesion provides convenience for some people, so they do not need to shop a la carte for various supplemental coverages. For others, it creates unappealing constraints. "I never wanted to go into HMO because you had to use their doctors," 98-year-old Clara told me when I asked if she had considered signing up for Medicare Advantage. "Maybe you don't care for them," Clara explained her thinking. "This way, now I have one doctor, and that's fine with me." She did not like the sense that she could be locked into someone else's health choices for her or treated by whichever doctor might be on duty.

Lillian, a part-time nurse who had turned 65 the year before we met, also objected to the notion of an HMO. "I wasn't even interested." She assumed services would be strictly limited, and she'd have little choice. "'We're going to manage it. We're going to tell you who you can go to. We've got a gatekeeper. We're going to cover your drugs but we're going to tell you which ones you can have.'"

More flexible Medigap or Medicare supplemental plans, offer partial additional coverage for nearly one-third (29%) of Medicare beneficiaries.[11] The average cost nationwide was just more than $1,700 per year, or $143 per month, though these costs vary by state and plan.[12]

Though almost one-third (30%) of Medicare beneficiaries get comprehensive or supplemental private plans via an employer's retiree benefits, most private plans are sold directly to individuals. Collectively, these older Americans earned private insurers $310 billion[13] in 2017. Thus, consumers 65 and over have a rare designation in health care: they are customers. Valuable customers. And, it turns out, the Medicare market works pretty well for them.

A WORKING MARKETPLACE OFFERING ABUNDANT CHOICE

For all that critics of government-sponsored insurance argue that overregulation will kill competition, Medicare shows that market forces can flourish in a highly regulated space.

Starting at age 65, Americans can go online each year to a functioning digital marketplace—Medicare.gov—to peruse and select from an array of comprehensive and supplemental private plans.

"They do have a really good website," Lillian described. "You can put your zip code in and put your other stuff in, and it will be able to pull up information on supplemental plans in your state, in your zip code, and the pharmaceutical plans. It's all there on the website, which is kind of amazing." This capability may not seem amazing; such online experiences are the norm in most other categories. In health insurance, though, Medicare.gov represents a dramatic transformation in the health insurance market. "You plug in things and it can actually give you all the costs."

Unlike many Americans who feel they must choose between unappealing health plan options—if they have any options at all[14]—Americans aged 65 and over can have an abundance of choice. For Medicare enrollees, choices are increasing. Nationwide, total available Medicare Advantage plans increased by almost 20%, and each Medicare beneficiary had an average of 24 plan choices from an average of 7 companies in 2019.[15] The vast majority (91%) of beneficiaries had a choice of 10 or more plans.[16] Almost everyone on Medicare (99%) has at least one Medicare Advantage or prescription plan available.[17]

Lillian chose from among 21 plan options. Both the number and dynamic nature of the options made it feel like the process of selecting an airplane ticket on a travel site. "You call and talk to somebody and they give you one price and then you check it online and it's another price. If you blink, it changes." Choosing flights can be overwhelming, but more options also make it more likely you'll find a choice that works for you.

Phyllis, Clara's daughter, is herself a retiree in her 70s with a Medicare Advantage plan, and she has been the appointed Medicare shopper for several elderly relatives, including her mother. "I don't think it takes me an hour now," Phyllis reflected on the selection process. "But when it first came out, it took me a very long time," more like four or five hours for each of three relatives she helped. She would gather the prescription information for each one—which drugs they take and at what doses, input the drug information, and sort through the different options. "The program will let you save the drugs, so unless there are changes, it's a snap."

Phyllis is organized and detail oriented, so she keeps printouts of the prior year's selection, digs them out of her paper files during open enrollment, and compares new options to the current plan. She can easily identify how the prices change year over year and what the best options really are. "You get a list of Part D insurers, usually in order of ascending cost. The premium might vary. The copay might vary. So, even though the website will tell you what your net cost is probably going to be for the year, there may be a feature of the insurance that you don't like, like higher copays or deductibles." The initial list of options might have eight or ten options and some are obviously not real options. Like shopping for an airline ticket, Phyllis said, "you don't even look at the ones that are $2,000 to go 200 miles. . . . The ones that are that far down are way more expensive. So, it's really more like three or four that are in the same ballpark. I think it's enough."

MULTIPLE AVENUES FOR PERSONAL SUPPORT

Not everyone has a Phyllis—an adult child capable and committed enough to help navigate these decisions, so Medicare also offers support. While enrollment support for individuals buying ACA plans has been eviscerated—with funding for navigators cut by 60% and advertising by 90%[18]—Medicare beneficiaries get a lot of attention. In addition to information and shopping options available at Medicare.gov, Medicare publishes a 100-plus page *Medicare & You* manual[19] and funds a national network of local enrollment counselors,[20] with an annual budget of approximately $50 million[21] (compared with $10 million[22] for Obamacare navigators in 2018).

Lillian explained the help available. "There is a bunch of written literature, and if that's too overwhelming for people, there are insurance agents that actually do sell Medicare supplemental plans. Of course, your premium's going to be higher because they've got to be paid for being able to hold the people's hands and walk them through this process."

In addition to private insurance agents who help consumers in support of their own financial incentives, the government funds volunteers to help beneficiaries navigate the system. "There are people that are really well trained in helping you. They're not going to be prejudiced towards one plan or the other, because they're not going to be making any money on what they're selling." Lillian herself had tapped into this assistance despite being a health care insider.

DELIVERING QUALITY AND VALUE

Private Medicare plans deliver high quality for relatively good value. Most enrollees choose private plans with high-quality ratings and extra benefits like dental and vision benefits not covered by traditional Medicare. Nearly three-quarters of Medicare Advantage members are in a plan rated four stars or higher (out of five) by the federal agency responsible for Medicare, and the majority get dental (62%), fitness (69%), and/or vision (77%) benefits.[23]

Phyllis described factoring quality into her recommendations for her mother Clara's supplemental prescription plan. "I used to look at the rating of the plans and the consumer service rating," she told me. "Some of them are quite bad, and that was a turn off. We definitely did not accept certain plans that had one star instead of three, four, or five." No amount of cost savings would make her choose a low-quality plan for her mother.

Ruth was also willing to pay more for a higher-quality plan. A retired social worker, she got supplemental insurance through her benefits as a school system retiree from Connecticut. "Last year I had a choice to change. I'm paying more to stay with this company that's been wonderful." (There's the word "wonderful" again.) Her current plan allows her to see a wide range of doctors, even out of state. "I can go to any place I want. I don't have to get it cleared." The unconstrained choice of one's own doctor was a powerful incentive to stay with that plan.

The new, cheaper alternative Ruth was offered had a bad reputation. "They sent a lot of stuff in the mail, which I read. Before you go to an emergency room, you need to get clearance from your insurance. . . . It was just a large company that I read a lot of negative things about. So, that was my main reason [for not switching]," Ruth explained.

It may be easier to pay more for higher-quality plans because Medicare costs have remained stable. Though plan costs can vary widely, average out-of-pocket costs cap out at just over $5,000 per year, and premiums for Medicare Advantage prescription drug plans—which only half of enrollees pay at all—have stayed nearly constant since 2012.[24] In fact, even as overall Medicare costs continue to rise, per person spending is slowing down. The rate of increase in per capita Medicare spending dropped in half, from 9% between 2000 and 2010 to 4.5% between 2010 and 2017.[25] Per person, Medicare spending increased by just about 1% per year between 2007 and 2016, less than the rate of inflation.[26]

Ruth's premium also went down, which she realized after she insisted on retrieving her statement and reading the exact numbers to me. "Does this make sense?" she asked. "Medical was $259 a month. And the new amount for this coming year is $238 a month." Ruth's choice to stay on the plan she was so happy with had cost more than if she had switched but less than it used to cost her. I'd call that a win.

SATISFIED CUSTOMERS

The health care system designed for older Americans—without question—is a more fair, equitable, and effective one than most other Americans experience. The federal government ensures near universal access to basic health coverage for Americans aged 65 and over, excluding only those who have not worked and paid Medicare taxes and did not have a spouse who worked and paid Medicare taxes for at least ten years.[27] Only 1.4% of Americans over 65 are uninsured, compared to approximately 9% overall.[28] Medicare benefits are mandated and robust, ensuring all Medicare beneficiaries have basic health coverage. Consumers with resources to afford additional coverage can choose supplemental plans and retain flexibility or buy fully managed comprehensive Medicare Advantage plans. Federal regulations standardize benefits and ensure coverage value, making it easier for consumers to trust what they're buying. Support exists to help people navigate a still-complex system, and costs have been stable, even declining in cases.

It's no wonder, then, that people over age 65 are the happiest of any age group with their health care. Per Gallup, nearly 90% of Americans aged 65 and older rate their health coverage as excellent or good, compared with the national average of 69%.[29]

Older consumers know how lucky they are, health-insurance-wise. "It's pretty wonderful coverage," Bernice described her Medicare supplemental plan, a federal government employee retiree benefit through her late husband. "Every year I think, 'What is the government going to do with this? And will they take it away?'" But her actual experience has been positive. "This year the premium went down $2.19. It's pretty exciting."

"I've been very fortunate," Howard reflected. Recently retired from a long career in television production, he had had employer-provided health insurance for decades, retiring around the time he became eligible for Medicare. A stint in the U.S. army and decades of military reserve service qualified him for supplemental coverage by Tricare for Life. "It's really been a blessing because I haven't had to deal with any of the issues of the Medicare Part D that most senior citizens these days struggle with, trying to figure out the best coverages and the intricacies of which form of Part D coverage is best for them." His military retiree benefits provide blanket coverage. "I don't give it a second thought."

Ruth similarly recognized, "I am lucky, in this country, very lucky to have the coverage that I do and I'm very aware of that. They haven't covered certain things but I can't complain really, given the present climate." Not only do many younger Americans have more difficulty navigating the system, many simply go without as much coverage or support as older Americans can access.

THE OTHER SIDE OF THE COIN

The upside of a functioning consumer market is that many people get what they need and want in that market. The downside is that people with fewer financial resources have fewer, if any, options. Shopping—theoretically open to anyone—can itself be a privilege. Even though Medicare presents a robust shopping opportunity for many older Americans, this consumer health insurance market leaves some older Americans behind. Not all Medicare beneficiaries are lucky enough to have retiree benefits or the means to buy private coverage. One in five Medicare beneficiaries, or six million people, have no supplemental coverage, leaving them completely exposed to coverage gaps.[30]

In fact, many older Americans face outright financial vulnerability. In 2017, nearly five million (9.2%) Americans aged 65 and older lived in poverty, earning less than $12,000 per year. Fifteen million (30.1%) had incomes less than 200% of the federal poverty level. By the more nuanced supplemental poverty measure, which accounts for geographic differences as well as financial resources and liabilities, almost half of older Americans could be considered poor.[31] Poverty rates increase with age and are higher for women (under supplemental poverty measure, 4 million women versus 2.7 million men), people of color, and people in relatively poor health.[32]

Older Americans are also more financially vulnerable than many of their peers around the world. In a global study, Americans over 65 had the highest rates of economic vulnerability—25%—of any country.[33] Brandeis University's Institute of Assets and Social Policy reported that one-third of senior households had no money left over or were in debt after paying essential expenses.[34]

This financial vulnerability spills directly into the health care arena. Nearly one-quarter (23%) of Americans 65 and older cite health care costs as the most important financial challenge facing their family, the top challenge by far for this age group.[35] Approximately 7.5 million Americans over 65 report being unable to pay for prescription medicines.[36] Researchers have found correlations between likelihood of depression or anxiety and higher out-of-pocket costs, lack of access to medications due to costs, and difficulty paying bills.[37]

Access to dental care is a particular challenge because Medicare offers no dental coverage. The majority of Americans over 65 have no dental insurance and almost half had not been to a dentist in the past year.[38] People between 50 and 64 do not tend to realize that dental care is not included in Medicare coverage,[39] leaving them less prepared for the lack of coverage. Overall, 10% of Medicare beneficiaries went without needed dental care due to cost barriers, which doubles to nearly 20% for those with incomes below 200% of the federal poverty level.[40] Two-thirds of people over 65 with incomes under $35,000 could not afford extensive dental care such as crowns, implants, or bridges.[41] More than a third of lower-income older Americans have no teeth at all.[42]

Not only are many older Americans financially vulnerable, the Medicare shopping experience does not work for everyone. For instance, the shopping tools require a sometimes-steep learning curve. Ralph, the retired executive in his 70s profiled in Chapter 6, said shopping on Medicare.gov was one of his most frustrating health care experiences. "I consider myself a reasonably intelligent individual, but I, in addition to a number of other people, have had tremendous difficulty negotiating the website. It's frustrating because I keep on thinking, 'I'm at least average intelligence, and I'm having problems with it.'"

He found himself tripped up by small details. "They're trying to make it as easy as possible, but every once in a while, they throw in these little ringers, or there's something wrong with the computer." Ralph had called the State Health Insurance Program, a support center to help Medicare beneficiaries navigate the system. "They train a whole bunch of volunteers, so when I was having all these problems, I called them up, and even they got screwed up on stuff, and they're the ones who were trained on what to do."

Ralph's struggles may reflect a natural phenomenon. Financial literacy appears to decline as people age. One study showed a clear decline on a standard financial literacy measure—without a similar decline in confidence—after age 60, across key demographic groups, attributed to age-related cognitive degradation.[43] Though not all decision-making skills decline with age,[44] older people made more financial mistakes than middle-aged subjects.[45]

In another study, the majority (56%) of older consumers had difficulty using comparative health plan information. The study authors cautioned against assuming market-based approaches will serve the older population well.[46] Whether or not that study—published in 2001—reflects increased consumer sophistication across age groups as technology has advanced since then, it still suggests that no matter how hard Medicare works to make its website and shopping platform easy to use, it probably can't make health insurance simple for everyone, especially those experiencing age-related cognitive decline.

WHAT CAN EVERYONE ELSE LEARN FROM MEDICARE AND ITS BENEFICIARIES?

Despite its imperfections, Medicare largely works for its beneficiaries. It provides choice, support, and financial protection—all at reasonable prices. To provide such a system to more Americans, voters could support policies and politicians that seek to expand Medicare's key market and regulatory features to more, if not all, Americans.

But that kind of reform faces uphill political struggles and may be a long way off if it ever arrives. In the meantime, we all might learn from older consumers how to become better health care shoppers or at least how to get more value from the health care options we have available. Here are six common themes I gleaned from the older people I interviewed:

1. Learn to navigate the system and tools available

Medicare.gov launched in 1998,[47] when some of the older people I interviewed were in their 70s and already on Medicare. Online shopping is now so obvious a norm young adults never operated in a world without it. Yet to older Americans—imprinted with the long history of the offline world—online marketplaces were a new way to shop.

Phyllis successfully mastered new tools and systems to navigate new insurance options for three elderly relatives and then for herself. This willingness to learn makes new options accessible and helps consumers capture value. It helps that Medicare.gov is a pretty good website, but older Americans who embrace new technologies model for everyone else the value and potential of learning and evolving.

2. Get and stay organized

The older consumers I interviewed tended to be extremely organized, likely a selection bias that led more organized people to schedule meetings with me. Still, this small and unscientific sample offers some useful lessons for other health care consumers, not to mention a note on aging well and remaining sharp and independent.

Ninety-eight-year-old Clara recited her monthly premium amounts to the penny for each of her supplemental plans. She told me her prescription plan premium was "$17.70 a month, that I know." Service for the monitor she wears around her neck costs "$38.13 every month," she also told me. "On the nose," Phyllis chimed in from the sideline. Clara writes the checks each month, so she knows.

Helen balances her checkbook each month to the penny.

When I asked Ruth if she had dental coverage, she said, "Oh God, I didn't know you were going to ask me this! It's gotten changed two or three times. Whatever it is, I've gone with it. I'm fairly organized so I've got files. I just pulled out dental." She had her files at the ready.

Others also offered to find the exact amount they pay in their files. Even though I explained I did not need the detail, some people made me wait while they retrieved the bill or explanation of benefits from their insurer, just as Ruth had. They retrieved such items from—or knew exactly where they were in—paper files: yes, paper files. Though today, many young people—and older ones who embrace Millennial culture—have gone paperless, these older people I met had a system. They kept their administrative lives in order. As difficult and for some impractical as it is to stay on top of health care and health insurance bills and policies and paperwork, those who can manage it seem in control, and less helpless, in health care purchasing.

3.   Ask questions

I met a group of older women at an assisted-living facility to talk to them about health care. Many of these women were in their 90s, and because we were in the Boston area—a health care hub—several had held professional roles in the field, as nurses or administrators. Whether informed by these experiences or by wisdom earned through life experience, or just a matter of their personalities, this group of health care consumers was among the most empowered I have ever encountered.

"When I grew up, a nurse had to stand when a doctor came into the room," one woman in her 90s explained. "We put them on a pedestal and wouldn't dare question them." Even educated and highly intelligent people did not question medical professionals. Doctors knew best. But one woman told me, "We have outgrown this, thank goodness!"

Some older Americans are still afraid to ask questions or challenge their health insurer, the government, or a hospital, for fear of retaliation or of being unable to get the care they need. Not these women. "I ask questions all the way along," a tiny 90-plus-year-old born in the United Kingdom told me from her wheelchair. "That is the key." She offered advice anyone could and should follow when a doctor or other clinician makes a recommendation. "Always ask, 'Is this covered by insurance?' and 'What would happen if I don't follow this recommendation?'" Despite her small stature, dignified accent, and diminished mobility, she spoke with confidence and authority, perhaps because of her career at a major teaching hospital. "It is very important to know the basics. It is, nowadays, a business. As in any business, you have to know your rights and duties." Just as you would not— or ought not—sign a legal document without reviewing it, she normalized the act of asking questions, even of authority figures. "There is nothing unusual about wanting to know the answer."

4.   Respect professionals, but think for yourself

"My overall approach at this point in my life is [that] I probably wouldn't treat most things that I might get," Ruth explained. At 85, she said, "my goal in life is not to live as long as I can. It's more about quality of life," which she defined by her financial stability, cognitive abilities, social connections, and overall independence.

Ruth's crystal-clear definition of her goals and priorities influenced her health care decisions. "I had breast cancer years ago. After a number of years, I stopped getting mammograms. If I were to get it back, I wouldn't have treated it. Things that need a lot of treatment, aggressive treatment, no, absolutely I would not do that." She conveyed her intentions to her doctors and her daughter, who serves as her health care proxy.

On another occasion, she saw a dermatologist when a rash she had did not get better on its own. The doctor insisted he do a full-body scan in order to be a "good dermatologist." On that scan, he found something on her back and suggested she get a biopsy. "I questioned him about it. 'Why?' and 'Would it kill me?'" They discussed her options, and he agreed it was fine not to test it, telling her to come back if it changed. "He heard me. And he didn't try to change my mind. And clearly I'm not dying from it or I think he would have [pushed his point of view on me]."

5. Self-advocate

Sam, an 83-year-old retired computer programmer, had recently fallen and hit his head. He had been admitted to the intensive care unit, even though he felt no discomfort, other than wanting to go home. I asked if he felt he had a say; could he use his voice and demand, or at least ask, to go home? "Theoretically I have a say," he told me. "But I would not go against them. I'm not—in this context—about to go against the medical opinion, because I respect the concern that it originates from."

But this general deference for physicians may be dissipating. For example, Ruth advocated for herself years earlier, when she noted a billing error. "I do read my bills and I was billed for something that wasn't true and I did call." She stood up for the right thing and never went back to that doctor, voting with her feet.

Lillian had a story of extreme self-advocacy, prior to her eligibility for Medicare, that likely influenced her behavior into her 60s. "I had major surgery and the insurance company went belly up. I was wicked tenacious, and I got specific people to talk to and I called every week. I sent letters and I complained to the attorney general in the state. And I am probably one of the only people that it actually finally paid all of my health care on the claim. It took two years to get all that money paid, but I didn't let go of it." Her self-advocacy paid off in material financial terms.

6. Partner with your doctors

Older consumers described long-term relationships with their doctors or other health care providers. "I had a wonderful doctor for many decades who retired a couple of years ago," Howard told me. "I trusted him completely. He was knowledgeable and kind and considerate. It couldn't have been better for me really. I was very sad when he retired."

He stayed with the clinic despite his doctor's retirement, since he had been happy there for decades.

Growing up in the United Kingdom, the diminutive former hospital professional described community doctors who were like friends. Another woman at the assisted-living facility who had grown up in Germany similarly described family doctors as friends of the family. "There were relationships."

Stanley, an 89-year-old retiree, told me about his doctor. "I have a wonderful physician. I've had him since the eighties." Stanley's friend—the doctor's brother-in-law—had recommended him, and Stanley had been one of this doctor's first patients. "He cares about me. He knows me intimately. He calls me on the phone. He takes my calls. He sees me immediately." Stanley's deep personal ties to his doctor yield easy access to his doctor.

These consumers described a level of longevity young adults seem not to have proclivity for, let alone time to have experienced. Compared with Millennials, almost half of whom do not even have a primary care doctor,[48] this older generation of patients may be anachronistic.* As health care complexity grows, and demands on physicians' time seems to exponentially increase, these relationships may fade with this passing generation. The emergence of Millennial-friendly options—from retail clinics and stand-alone urgent-care centers to virtual visits using online platforms—improve on convenience, timeliness, and price transparency[49] but will not deliver consistency or long-term relationships.

It's not just patients who benefit from long-term, authentic clinical relationships. Doctors do too. "Fundamentally, medicine is about relationships," Suzanne Koven, MD, told me. A practicing internist showcased in Chapter 8, Koven described the importance of developing patient-doctor relationships. "It's the most fun and gratifying part of medicine for me."

In a large survey of physicians nationwide, the majority (88%) reported positive relationships with patients and 87% reported that the most gratifying aspect of being a doctor is interacting with and helping patients.[50] Relationships matter to all involved.

MEDICARE FOR MORE

Politics aside, Medicare is a health system worth emulating. In its current form, Medicare offers private-sector competition to expand consumer

---

* Only 12% of people over 65 do not have a PCP (*Source:* https://www.kff.org/other/slide/one-fourth-of-adults-and-nearly-half-of-adults-under-30-dont-have-a-primary-care-doctor/).

choice and value, and a consumer-friendly online marketplace on which consumers pursue their own choices. It also provides standard benefits, consumer protections, and support to help consumers make good decisions for themselves.

Whether policy makers would expand Medicare to more Americans is a wide open question. Doing so would increase the role of government in American health insurance. It may add substantial cost to the federal budget, though some experts project long-term savings from even the most extreme single-payer designs.[51]

Expanding Medicare would provide a much-needed safety net for millions of uninsured Americans—a progressive dream—while also enabling a larger private market. Americans would more squarely play a role conservatives should love: health care shopper. Expanding consumer choices built on a system that already works for millions of consumers could mean new access to a true health care market for all Americans.

Whether or until such reforms happen, Americans can still benefit from the example older consumers are setting. They're taking advantage of a system designed to help and support them in getting the care they need. They're investing in long-term relationships with trusted physicians. And they're evaluating their coverage options and making decisions—actively or passively—to meet their needs.

16

Attention Shoppers!

How to move the health care market with your wallet

I am sitting alone in my car in the mall parking lot. Like my dad, who throughout my childhood would arrive home but sit in the car until whatever NPR story he was listening to had finished, I do not want to go in yet.

I am here to return a dress to Nordstrom. It is an extra dress. It is long and pretty, and I like it. I had bought it just in case I changed my mind about the dress I intended to wear to my big event or in case I could come up with another occasion for it. But I did not wear it and have not come up with any new ideas to justify the purchase. I have responsibly decided I don't need an extra dress and trekked out to the suburbs to return it.

On the radio, though, is the TED Radio Hour,[1] featuring Adora Svitak, who was 12 years old when she gave a TED talk: "What adults can learn from kids."[2] Svitak beseeches adults not to underestimate children and reminds adults that they, too, once yearned to be listened to and respected.

"Our inherent wisdom doesn't have to be insider's knowledge," she says. She reframes wide-eyed, naive thinking—usually derided as childish—into a wiser, more-expansive lens. "Our audacity to imagine helps push the boundaries of possibility."

Whereas adults' experience, appreciation of complexity, and knowledge of past failures cramp their creativity, kids are less informed about how hard things might be. "We kids aren't hampered as much when it comes to thinking about reasons why not to do things," this young sage says. "And that's a good thing because in order to make anything a reality, you have to dream about it first."

This 12-year-old unknowingly summarizes the biggest obstacles to change in the U.S. health care system: lack of audacity to imagine new possibilities and an over-abundance of knowledge of past failures. Paralyzed by keen understanding of intricacies and complexities of the system, the system's adults—health care insiders and experts—know too much about how difficult change is to achieve.

Adora Svitak perfectly articulates what consumers can do for health care. Consumers using the system and discovering its inadequacies are the kids in this situation. And they—we—know enough to ask questions, to expect better, and to challenge the impossibility of transformation.

Health care in America is a notoriously slow-moving industry. Large bureaucracies rule both the public and private sectors. Technological complexities both spur clinical innovations and weigh down large organizations. Cultural norms and traditions firmly grasp doctors and patients alike. Huge amounts of money are at stake, and incumbent players often strongly resist change. Even change agents—innovators, entrepreneurs, and creative scholars—usually start by biting off only one, seemingly attackable problem, overwhelmed by the enormity and interconnectedness of the problems in American health care. Change is, by necessity, incremental and can feel painfully slow and insufficient.

A whole literature exists on why the U.S. health care system is costly, inefficient, and broken. Scholars study the problems. Industry conferences gather executives to discuss solutions. Huge amounts of capital are invested in search of profits from disrupting the status quo.

Consumers are too often overlooked in these efforts, dismissed as unimportant in the financial equation. The average consumer does not matter that much in economic terms. Just as many potential voters don't participate in American democracy, claiming no one vote swings an election, consumers often feel insignificant and helpless to change the system.

But many U.S. elections—at all levels of government—have turned on exceedingly small margins. Single votes accumulate and together matter a lot. So it is with consumers in health care.

Consumers who shared their stories with me described confusion, anger, immense frustration, and apathy about their health care system encounters. Almost no one I met felt like an expert or felt competent in health care. "I know nothing about health care, but I'm happy to talk to you," many people said.

And they did know something about health care—every last one. In fact, they had expertise in some of the most important aspects of health care: how they felt about and experienced it, what they understood and did not understand about it, and what mattered most to them. Consumers' own experiences, priorities, and preferences are, in fact, foundational ingredients to reforming the U.S. health care system, if the goal is to make the system more responsive to consumers.

Here, in summary, is what I learned from their stories:

- There are a range of health care consumers, as there are in any product category—we should recognize different types of consumers with different needs and preferences.

- There are many different aspects to shopping involving individual motivations, preferences, and priorities—we should recognize shopping as the complex and legitimate process it is.

- Health care organizations and regulators often block consumer shopping behavior—we should recognize that they could do much more to make health care shopping substantially easier and more productive and we should demand that they do.

- Some people are already trying to shop in health care settings, contrary to economics dogma, yet they meet with numerous obstacles—we should recognize, encourage, and enable consumer shopping behaviors.

Thus, it is time for consumers to shift collective expectations and behaviors when buying health care services and coverage. Despite the diversity in shopper types, all health care consumers are entitled to certain fundamental expectations—such as to be heard, respected, and ultimately, treated as an important customer who deserves more value for our health care spending. Those expectations include the following:

1. **Price tags:** We should know what things cost before we pay, and prices should make sense relative to the value we receive. The industry needs to simplify underlying billing practices to make consumer-grade transparency and clarity a reality and develop competencies to proactively discuss costs with consumers (Chapter 5).

2. **Clarity:** We should understand what we're buying when we shop for health insurance. Insurers should simplify products and how those products are presented so consumers can effectively compare and make informed decisions when choosing and using benefits. Health plans, health professionals, and regulators should speak our language, avoid jargon, and authentically communicate with consumers (Chapters 11, 12, and 13).

3. **Quality:** We should define quality on our own terms and be able to choose providers based on what matters most to us. Health plans, providers, and accrediting bodies should give credence to consumer measures of quality and develop meaningful ways to quantify those values (Chapter 9).

4. **Service:** We should be treated as the customer, with our own needs and preferences, and recognized for our role in paying at least part of the bill. Clinicians, hospitals, and health plans should recognize that consumers' share of health care costs make us worthy of attention, care, respect, and accommodation (Chapters 2 and 4).

5. **Value:** We should get what we pay for, negotiate when we don't, and hold providers and health plans accountable to us for results. Insurers need to provide real value and enable, instead of deter, consumers from using benefits to which they are entitled (Chapters 6 and 13).

6. **Respect:** We should be treated with respect, partnership, and care. We should feel heard and feel that our concerns are taken seriously. Doctors and other clinicians should listen to consumers, take seriously consumer concerns and preferences, and recognize consumer expertise on our own bodies. Health care industry leaders should design and implement systems that enable genuine choice and value, with appropriate support for consumer decision-making. Health care providers should be our partners in care, recognizing we are whole people (Chapters 8 and 15).

7. **Assistance:** We should not be left alone to navigate our health care journeys at our most vulnerable or exasperated moments. Health plans and providers should assign staff to serve as points of accountability and take responsibility for issue resolution rather than unduly burdening consumers with navigating corporate disputes (Chapter 7).

8. **Portability:** We should not lose our health benefits when we need them most. Policy makers must protect and expand access to coverage outside of employment to allow career flexibility and freedom to pursue professional passions, while enabling modern labor market developments (Chapter 10).

9. **Dental care:** Our teeth should be recognized as integral parts of our bodies. Everyone has teeth and it should not be a privilege to care for them. Dentistry and medicine need to start working together to recognize, and behave as if, oral health is part of overall health (Chapter 14).

10. **Mental health:** We should have equal access to mental health care and be able to get care critical to overall health and well-being. Health insurers should recognize the value of mental health care to overall

health and well-being and create conditions that do not leave mental health clinicians feeling forced to opt out of the insurance system. At the same time, health care leaders should learn from mental health's price transparency and consumer empowerment (Chapter 3).

To make this consumer-oriented vision of the U.S. health care system a reality, health plans, health care providers, and regulators need to authentically put consumers in the center of their actions. They need to adopt consumer definitions of clarity, quality, and value. They must stop hiding behind bureaucracy and the legacy of complicating factors. They need to acknowledge the importance of consumers in the system and begin to ask about, listen for, and respond to consumer concerns and preferences.

Most important, consumers must demand these changes. Consumers should demand to be recognized as health care purchasers. Consumers who are recognized as customers are more likely to be treated as the true center of their health care decisions. To demand such change, we must first imagine it and believe that we deserve it. As Adora Svitak urges, we must have the audacity to imagine ourselves as health care consumers, worthy of consumer-grade experiences, information, and options. As she might put it, by imagining such a role for ourselves, we can "push the boundaries of possibility."

Becoming an empowered health care consumer, one who contributes to a movement of change in U.S. health care, requires adopting a mind-set befitting of a health care *customer*. This mind-set boils down to three fundamental elements, simple yet hard to implement.

First, health care consumers must engage in *inquiry*. We must ask questions. Why? What does this cost? What are my options? Finding one's voice is critical to getting the answers consumers need in order to make health care decisions. "There is nothing unusual about wanting to know the answer," the older British woman introduced in Chapter 15 told me. In fact, it's a bit crazy for anyone to expect consumers to make decisions without asking—and getting satisfactory answers—to all manner of questions.

Second, health care consumers must engage in *advocacy*. We must stand up for ourselves, whether to make sure a doctor hears our full story, as we want to tell it, or to fight erroneous medical bills or insurance denials. Self-advocacy is about more than what you can get as an individual. That is important, too. But the higher-order importance of your efforts to extract value for yourself is that others will benefit, too. Alone, any single effort may not yield change, rationality, or fairness. But together, engagement can force needed changes in health care. So even if you might not be moved to fight for yourself, do your part to fight your individual case on behalf of us all.

Finally, health care consumers must adopt a sense of *ownership*. We must engage in health care decisions as if we were spending our own money—because we are. Painful as it can be, we should pay attention, build competency, and act as if our decisions have consequences. They do. For us and everyone else. When we hold a doctor's office accountable for an erroneous bill, or when we dispute an insurance company denial, or even just call for clarification, we are taking small steps that show these entities we are paying attention. We are watching. And we will hold them accountable. They'll do a better job for us as a result, maybe not right away or because of one phone call. But a pattern, trend, or even wave of consumer engagement will get their attention.

Malaz Boustani from the Indiana University School of Medicine, who shared his views on health care quality in Chapter 9, summed up how best to transform American health care: "We need to empower the consumer to revolt. And take back their power." Boustani urges consumers to "become customers, and fight and choose and punish the health care system that does not provide safe, high-reliability, personalized and evidence-based services," which should include high-value health care and coverage.

"Wouldn't it be lovely if someone started a revolution?" my friend and long-time political activist suggested when I described this book. Yes, someone should do that. Let's make it us.

So, knock on this door. Bang on it, even. It may not open at first or for any one person knocking. But keep knocking. Each knock on the door helps open it a crack, and once enough consumers insist on opening the door, the door will open.

Notes

INTRODUCTION

1. Robin A. Cohen, Emily P. Terlizzi, and Michael E. Martinez, "Health Insurance Coverage: Early Release of Estimates from the National Health Interview Survey, 2018," Division of Health Interview Statistics, National Center for Health Statistics, released May 2019, https://www.cdc.gov/nchs/data/nhis/earlyrelease/insur201905.pdf.

2. Sara R. Collins, Munira Z. Gunja, and Michelle M. Doty, "How Well Does Insurance Coverage Protect Consumers from Health Care Costs?" The Commonwealth Fund, October 2017, https://www.commonwealth fund.org/sites/default/files/documents/___media_files_publications_ issue_brief_2017_oct_collins_underinsured_biennial_ib.pdf.

3. https://data.worldbank.org/country/Indonesia.

4. Sara R. Collins, Herman K. Bhupal, and Michelle M. Doty, "Health Insurance Coverage Eight Years after the ACA," The Commonwealth Fund, February 7, 2019, https://www.commonwealthfund.org/publica tions/issue-briefs/2019/feb/health-insurance-coverage-eight-years-after-aca.

5. Gary Claxton, Matthew Rae, Michelle Long, Anthony Damico, Gregory Young, Daniel McDermott, and Heidi Whitmore, "Employer Health Benefits 2019 Annual Survey," Kaiser Family Foundation, 2019, http://files.kff.org/attachment/Report-Employer-Health-Benefits-Annual-Survey-2019.

6. Kenneth J. Arrow, "Uncertainty and the Welfare Economics of Medical Care," *The American Economic Review* 53, no. 5 (1963): 941–73.

7. Ibid.

8. Atul Gawande, "The Cost Conundrum," *The New Yorker* 85, no. 16 (2009).

9. Jay Greene and Abha Bhattarai, "Attention, Walmart Executives: Amazon's Coming after Your Low-Income Shoppers," *The Washington Post*, June 18, 2019, https://www.washingtonpost.com/technology/2019/06/18/amazons-growing-prime-focus-americas-poor/.

10. Maria LaMagna, "Jeff Bezos Really Wants Low-Income Consumers to Subscribe to Amazon Prime," *MarketWatch*, April 19, 2018, https://www.marketwatch.com/story/amazon-has-made-a-point-of-targeting-low-income-customers-2018-01-26.

11. CBN, "The Surprising Purchasing Power of Low-Income Consumers: Why Amazon (and Other Smart Businesses) Won't Ignore This Important Market," *Cascade Business News*, June 29, 2017, http://cascadebusnews.com/surprising-purchasing-power-low-income-consumers-amazon-smart-businesses-wont-ignore-important-market/.

CHAPTER 1

1. Alexandra Talty, "Yes, Americans Can Still Travel to Cuba," *Forbes*, April 23, 2018, https://www.forbes.com/sites/alexandratalty/2018/04/23/yes-you-can-still-travel-to-cuba.

2. Alexandra Talty, "Cuba to Welcome 5 Million Visitors in 2019," *Forbes*, February 7, 2019, https://www.forbes.com/sites/alexandratalty/2019/02/07/cuba-to-welcome-5-million-visitors-in-2019.

3. Richard E. Feinberg and Richard S. Newfarmer, "Tourism in Cuba: Riding the Wave toward Sustainable Prosperity," Brookings Institution Report, December 2, 2016, https://www.brookings.edu/research/tourism-in-cuba/.

4. John Andrew Gustavsen, "Tension under the Sun: Tourism and Identity in Cuba, 1945–2007" (Dissertation, University of Miami, 2009), 298, https://scholarlyrepository.miami.edu/oa_dissertations/298.

5. Deborah Cohen, "Chain Reaction," *Indianapolis Monthly*, August 2008, 89–99.

6. Jamie Ballard and Amanda Garrity, "30 Celebrities You Didn't Know Were Vegan," *Good Housekeeping*, December 20, 2018, https://www.goodhousekeeping.com/life/g5186/vegan-celebrities/.

7. Dkellerm, "Sasquatch Music Festival 2009—Guy Starts Dance Party," uploaded May 26, 2009, YouTube video, 3:05, https://www.youtube.com/watch?v=GA8z7f7a2Pk.

8. Derek Sivers, "First Follower: Leadership Lessons from Dancing Guy," uploaded February 11, 2010, YouTube video, https://www.youtube.com/watch?v=fW8amMCVAJQ.

9. Janet Forgrieve, "The Growing Acceptance of Veganism," *Forbes*, November 2, 2018, https://www.forbes.com/sites/janetforgrieve/2018/11/02/picturing-a-kindler-gentler-world-vegan-month.

10.   The Good Food Institute, "Plant-Based Market Overview," The Good Food Institute, based on data released July 16, 2019, https://www.gfi .org/marketresearch.

11. Michelle Feinberg, "The Best Vegan-Friendly Restaurants to Visit with Your Not-Yet-Vegan Family," PETA, March 15, 2019, https://www .peta.org/living/food/best-vegan-friendly-restaurants-for-nonvegan-family/.

12. Caroline Shannon-Karasik, "16 Fast-Food Orders That Actually Are Vegan," *Women's Health*, June 20, 2019, https://www.womenshealthmag .com/food/a22594071/best-vegan-fast-food/.

13. Forgrieve, "The Growing Acceptance of Veganism."

14. Jeanine Bentley, "Per Capita Availability of Chicken Higher Than That of Beef," Economic Research Service, United States Department of Agriculture, last updated August 28, 2019, https://www.ers.usda.gov/data-products/chart-gallery/gallery/chart-detail/?chartId=58312.

15. Zachary Crockett, "The Worst Sales Promotion in History," *The Hustle*, August 10, 2019, https://thehustle.co/the-worst-sales-promotion-in-history/.

16. Andrew Tonner, "7 Sam Walton Quotes You Should Read Right Now," The Motley Fool, September 8, 2016, https://www.fool.com/ investing/2016/09/08/7-sam-walton-quotes-you-should-read-right-now .aspx.

CHAPTER 2

1. Diana Farrell and Fiona Greig, "Paying Out-of-Pocket: The Health-care Spending of 2 Million US Families," JP Morgan Chase Institute, September 2009, https://www.jpmorganchase.com/content/dam/jpmorgan chase/en/legacy/corporate/institute/document/institute-healthcare.pdf.

2. Matthew Rae, Rebecca Copeland, and Cynthia Cox, "Tracking the Rise in Premium Contributions and Cost-Sharing for Families with Large Employer Coverage," Kaiser Family Foundation Briefs, August 14, 2019, https://www.healthsystemtracker.org/brief/tracking-the-rise-in-premium-contributions-and-cost-sharing-for-families-with-large-employer-coverage/.

3. Craig J. Shearman, "2018 Holiday Sales Grew 2.9 Percent amid Tur-moil over Trade Policy and Delay in Data Collection," National Retail Fed-eration, February 14, 2019, https://nrf.com/media-center/press-releases/ 2018-holiday-sales-grew-29-percent-amid-turmoil-over-trade-policy-and.

4. Erica B. Levy, "HMS's 'New Pathway' Curriculum Copied at Other Schools," *The Harvard Crimson*, April 6, 1999, https://www.thecrimson .com/article/1999/4/6/hmss-new-pathway-curriculum-copied-at/.

5. Zoë Slote Morris, Steven Wooding, and Jonathan Grant, "The Answer Is 17 Years, What Is the Question: Understanding Time Lags in

Translational Research," *Journal of the Royal Society of Medicine* 104, no. 12 (2011): 510–20.

6. David Schleifer, Rebecca Silliman, and Chloe Rinehart, "Still Searching: How People Use Health Care Price Information in the United States," Public Agenda, April 2017, https://nyshealthfoundation.org/wp-content/uploads/2017/11/how-people-use-health-care-price-information-brief.pdf.

7. Phil Galewitz, "Doctors Slow to Adopt Tech Tools That Might Save Patients Money on Drugs," WBUR.org, July 5, 2019, https://www.wbur.org/npr/738283044/doctors-slow-to-adopt-tech-tools-that-might-save-patients-money-on-drugs.

8. Katrin Starcke and Mattias Brand, "Decision Making under Stress: A Selective Review," *Neuroscience and Biobehavioral Reviews* 36, no. 4 (2012): 1228–48.

9. Saurabh Bhargava, George Loewenstein, and Justin Sydnor, "Do Individuals Make Sensible Health Insurance Decisions? Evidence from a Menu with Dominated Options" (Working Paper No. 21160, National Bureau of Economic Research, May 2015).

10. www.venrock.com/teeaammember/bob-kocher.

11. Schleifer, Silliman, and Rinehart, "Still Searching."

12. David Mikkelson, "Nordstrom Tire Return: Did a Man Get a Refund for a Snow Tire from Nordstrom, a Store That Doesn't Sell Tires?" Snopes, updated April 25, 2011, https://www.snopes.com/fact-check/return-to-spender/.

13. Godwin-Charles Ogbeide, "Hospitality Intelligence: Evolution, Definition and Dimensions," *Events and Tourism Review* 2, no. 1 (2019): 1–20.

CHAPTER 3

1. Tara F. Bishop, Matthew J. Press, Salomeh Keyhani, and Harold Alan Pincus, "Acceptance of Insurance by Psychiatrists and the Implications for Access to Mental Health Care," *JAMA Psychiatry* 71, no. 2 (2014): 176–81.

2. Shefali Luthra, "Biden Calling ACA a 'Breakthrough' for Mental Health Parity Only Highlights Gaps," *Kaiser Health News*, July 11, 2019, https://khn.org/news/joe-biden-mental-health-parity-fact-check.

3. "The Doctor Is Out: Continuing Disparities in Access to Mental and Physical Health Care," National Alliance on Mental Illness, November 2017, https://www.nami.org/About-NAMI/Publications-Reports/Public-Policy-Reports/The-Doctor-is-Out/DoctorIsOut.pdf.

4. Ibid.

5. Thomas G. Mcguire and Jeanne Miranda, "New Evidence Regarding Racial and Ethnic Disparities in Mental Health: Policy Implications," *Health Affairs* 27, no. 2 (2008): 393–403.

6. Rabah Kamal, "What Are the Current Costs and Outcomes Related to Mental Health and Substance Use Disorders?" Kaiser Family Foundation Chart Collections, July 31, 2017, https://www.healthsystemtracker.org/chart-collection/current-costs-outcomes-related-mental-health-substance-abuse-disorders/#item-nine-percent-adults-suicidal-thoughts-report-using-illicit-drug.

7. Ibid.

8. "Spending on Disease Treatment," Peterson-Kaiser Health System Tracker, https://www.healthsystemtracker.org/indicator/spending/spending-disease-treatment/.

9. Substance Abuse and Mental Health Services Administration, Projections of National Expenditures for Treatment of Mental and Substance Use Disorders, 2010–2020, HHS Publication No. SMA-14-4883, 2014.

10. Charles Roehrig, "Mental Disorders Top the List of the Most Costly Conditions in the United States: $201 Billion," *Health Affairs* 35, no. 6 (2016): 1130–35.

11. Stephen P. Melek, Douglas T. Norris, Jordan Paulus, Katherine Matthews, Alexandra Weaver, and Stoddard Davenport, "Potential Economic Impact of Integrated Medical-Behavioral Healthcare," Milliman Research Report, January 2018, https://www.psychiatry.org/File%20Library/Psychiatrists/Practice/Professional-Topics/Integrated-Care/Milliman-Report-Economic-Impact-Integrated-Implications-Psychiatry.pdf.

12. Ibid.

13. Ibid.

14. Bruce Japsen, "Psychiatrist Shortage Escalates as U.S. Mental Health Needs Grow," *Forbes*, February 25, 2018, https://www.forbes.com/sites/brucejapsen/2018/02/25/psychiatrist-shortage-escalates-as-u-s-mental-health-needs-grow.

15. Larry R. Faulkner, Dorthea Juul, Naleen Andrade, Beth Ann Brooks, Christopher C. Colenda, Robert Guynn, David Mrazek, Victor Reus, Barbara Schneidman, and Kailie Shaw, "Recent Trends in American Board of Psychiatry and Neurology Psychiatric Subspecialties," *Academic Psychiatry* 35, no. 1 (2011): 35–39.

16. Stacy Weiner, "Addressing the Escalating Psychiatrist Shortage," AAMC News, February 13, 2018, https://news.aamc.org/patient-care/article/addressing-escalating-psychiatrist-shortage/.

17. "2019 Update: The Complexities of Physician Supply and Demand: Projections from 2017 to 2032," Association of American Medical Colleges, April 2019, https://aamc-black.global.ssl.fastly.net/production/media/filer_public/31/13/3113ee5c-a038-4c16-89af-294a69826650/2019_update_-_the_complexities_of_physician_supply_and_demand_-_projections_from_2017-2032.pdf.

18. Ibid.

19. "Mental Health Care Health Professional Shortage Areas (HPSAs)," State Health Facts, *Kaiser Health News,* as of December 31, 2018, https://www.kff.org/other/state-indicator/mental-health-care-health-professional-shortage-areas-hpsas/.

20. Ibid.

21. Mcguire and Miranda, "New Evidence Regarding Racial and Ethnic Disparities in Mental Health."

22. Sarah Grisham, "Medscape Physician Compensation Report 2017," Medscape, April 5, 2017, https://www.medscape.com/slideshow/compensation-2017-overview-6008547#4.

23. AAMC, Content Documentation in Required Courses and Elective Courses, AAMC, 2019, https://www.aamc.org/data-reports/curriculum-reports/interactive-data/content-documentation-required-courses-and-elective-courses.

CHAPTER 4

1. Diana Farrell and Fiona Greig, "Paying Out-of-Pocket: The Healthcare Spending of 2 Million U.S. Families," JP Morgan Chase Institute, September 2009, https://www.jpmorganchase.com/content/dam/jpmorganchase/en/legacy/corporate/institute/document/institute-healthcare.pdf.

2. Matthew Rae, Rebecca Copeland, and Cynthia Cox, "Tracking the Rise in Premium Contributions and Cost-Sharing for Families with Large Employer Coverage," Kaiser Family Foundation Briefs, August 14, 2019, https://www.healthsystemtracker.org/brief/tracking-the-rise-in-premium-contributions-and-cost-sharing-for-families-with-large-employer-coverage/.

3. Carrie Marie Schneider, "Psychographic Consumer Profiling," Glasstire, February 6, 2013, https://glasstire.com/2013/02/06/psychographic-consumer-profiling/.

4. Steve King, "What Kind of Traveller Are You?" *Condé Nast Traveler,* https://www.cntraveller.com/gallery/10-types-that-travel.

5. Seymour H. Fine, "Toward a Theory of Segmentation by Objectives in Social Marketing," *Journal of Consumer Research* 7, no. 1 (1980): 1–13.

6. "The U.S. Health Care Market: A Strategic View of Consumer Segmentation," Deloitte Center for Health Solutions, 2012, https://www2.deloitte.com/content/dam/Deloitte/us/Documents/life-sciences-health-care/us-lshc-health-care-market-consumer-segmentation.pdf.

7. "Psychographic Segmentation and the Healthcare Consumer," c2b solutions, 2017, https://www.c2bsolutions.com/psychographic-segmentation.

8. Christopher C. Duke, Wendy D. Lynch, Brad Smith, and Julie Winstanley, "Validity of a New Patient Engagement Measure: The Altarum Consumer Engagement (ACE) Measure™," *Patient-Centered Outcomes Research* 8, no. 6 (2015): 559–68.

9. Carl M. Cannon, "Poll: 'Medicare for All' Support Is High—But Complicated," RealClear Politics, May 15, 2019, https://www.realclearpoli tics.com/articles/2019/05/15/poll_medicare_for_all_support_is_high__ but_complicated_140327.html.

10. Deborah Gordon, "How Health Care Voters May Surprise Us," RealClear Politics, May 17, 2019, https://www.realclearpolitics.com/ 2019/05/17/how_health_care_voters_may_surprise_us_475069.html.

11. Ibid.

12. Justin McCarthy, "Most Americans Still Rate Their Healthcare Quite Positively," Gallup, December 7, 2018, https://news.gallup.com/ poll/245195/americans-rate-healthcare-quite-positively.aspx.

CHAPTER 5

1. Vineet Arora, Christopher Moriates, and Neel Shah, "The Challenge of Understanding Health Care Costs and Charges," *AMA Journal of Ethics* 17, no. 11 (2015): 1046–52.

2. Will Kenton, "Activity Based Costing (ABC)," Investopedia, August 23, 2019, https://www.investopedia.com/terms/a/abc.asp.

3. Australian Medical Association Limited, ABN 37 008 426 793, Position Statement on Informed Financial Consent (Australian Medical Association, 2015).

4. "AHIA's Position Paper on Informed Financial Consent (IFC)," Private Healthcare, Australia, March 2, 2006, https://www.privatehealth careaustralia.org.au/ahias-position-paper-on-informed-financial-consentifc/.

5. "Quarterly Private Health Insurance Statistics March 2019," Australian Prudential Regulation Authority, May 21, 2019, https://www.apra .gov.au/sites/default/files/quarterly_private_health_insurance_statis tics_-_march_2019.pdf.

6. T. R. Reid, *The Healing of America: A Global Quest for Better, Cheaper, and Fairer Health Care* (New York: Penguin Press, 2009), p. 54.

7. "Fee Benchmarks and Bill Amount Information," Ministry of Health Singapore, https://www.moh.gov.sg/cost-financing/fee-benchmarks-and-bill-amount-information.

8. "Fiscal Year (FY) 2019 Medicare Hospital Inpatient Prospective Payment System (IPPS) and Long-Term Acute Care Hospital (LTCH) Prospective Payment System Final Rule (CMS-1694-F)," CMS Newsroom, August 2, 2018, https://www.cms.gov/newsroom/fact-sheets/fiscal-year-fy-2019-medi care-hospital-inpatient-prospective-payment-system-ipps-and-long-term-acute-0.

9. Barbara Anthony and Scott Haller, "Massachusetts Hospitals Score Poorly on Price Transparency . . . Again," White Paper No. 167, Pioneer Institute, April 2017.

10. "Chapter 224: An Act Improving the Quality of Health Care and Reducing Costs through Increased Transparency, Efficiency, and Innovation," the 191st General Court of the Commonwealth of Massachusetts, approved August 6, 2012, https://malegislature.gov/Laws/SessionLaws/Acts/2012/Chapter224.

11. François de Brantes, Suzanne Delbanco, Erin Butto, Karina Patino-Mazmanian, and Lea Tessitore, "Price Transparency and Physician Quality Report Card 2017," Altarum and Catalyst for Payment Reform, November 8, 2017, https://altarum.org/sites/default/files/uploaded-publi cation-files/2017%20Price%20Transparency%20and%20Physician%20 Quality%20Report%20Card_0.pdf.

12. Ibid.

13. Christopher Whaley, Jennifer Schneider Chafen, Sophie Pinkard, Gabriella Kellerman, Dena Bravata, Robert Kocher, and Neeraj Sood, "Association between Availability of Health Service Prices and Payments for These Services," *JAMA* 312, no. 16 (2014): 1670–76.

14. Zarek C. Brot-Goldberg, Amitabh Chandra, Benjamin R. Handel, and Jonathan T. Kolstad, "What Does a Deductible Do? The Impact of Cost-Sharing on Health Care Prices, Quantities, and Spending Dynamics," *The Quarterly Journal of Economics* 132, no. 3 (2017): 1261–318.

15. Neeraj Sood, Zachary Wagner, Peter Huckfeldt, and Amelia Haviland, "Price-Shopping in Consumer-Directed Health Plans," *Forum for Health Economics & Policy* 16, no. 1 (2013): 1–19.

16. Sunita Desai, Laura A. Hatfield, Andrew L. Hicks, Michael E. Chernew, and Ateev Mehrotra, "Association between Availability of a Price Transparency Tool and Outpatient Spending," *JAMA* 315, no. 17 (2016): 1874–81.

17. Ateev Mehrotra, Katie M. Dean, Anna D. Sinaiko, and Neeraj Sood, "Americans Support Price Shopping for Health Care, But Few Actually Seek out Price Information," *Health Affairs* 36, no. 8 (2017): 1392–400.

18. Sunita Desai, Laura A. Hatfield, Andrew L. Hicks, Michael E. Chernew, and Ateev Mehrotra, "Association between Availability of a Price Transparency Tool and Outpatient Spending," *JAMA* 315, no. 17 (2016): 1874–81.

19. Ha Tu and Rebecca Gourevitch, "Moving Markets: Lessons from New Hampshire's Health Care Price Transparency Experiment," IDEAS Working Paper Series from RePEc, April 2014, https://www.chcf.org/wp-content/uploads/2017/12/PDF-MovingMarketsNewHampshire.pdf.

20. Chapin White and Megan Eguchi, "Reference Pricing: A Small Piece of the Health Care Price and Quality Puzzle," *Medical Benefits* 31, no. 23 (December 15, 2014): 4–5.

21. Amanda Frost and David Newman, "Spending on Shoppable Services in Health Care," Health Care Cost Institute Issue Brief No. 11, 2016, https://healthcostinstitute.org/research/publications/hcci-research/entry/spending-on-shoppable-services-in-health-care.

22. Ibid.

23. Phil Galewitz, "Doctors Slow to Adopt Tech Tools That Might Save Patients Money On Drugs," WBUR.org, July 5, 2019, https://www.wbur.org/npr/738283044/doctors-slow-to-adopt-tech-tools-that-might-save-patients-money-on-drugs.

24. "Fiscal Year (FY) 2019 Medicare Hospital Inpatient Prospective Payment System (IPPS)."

25. Anne Quito and Amanda Shendruk, "U.S. Hospitals Are Now Required by Law to Post Prices Online. Good Luck Finding Them," Quartz, January 15, 2019, https://qz.com/1518545/price-lists-for-the-115-biggest-us-hospitals-new-transparency-law/.

26. Christopher Moriates, Krishan Soni, Andrew Lai, and Sumant Ranji, "The Value in the Evidence: Teaching Residents to 'Choose Wisely,'" *JAMA Internal Medicine* 173, no. 4 (2013): 1–3.

27. AAMC, Content Documentation in Required Courses and Elective Courses, 2019, https://www.aamc.org/data-reports/curriculum-reports/interactive-data/content-documentation-required-courses-and-elective-courses.

28. Deborah Gordon, Gwendolyn Lee, Akshaya Kannan, and Roy Perlis, "A National Survey of U.S. Medical Students' Training and Attitudes Regarding Patient Financial Discussions." Manuscript in review.

29. Emmy Ganos, Katherine Steinberg, Joshua Seidman, Domitilla Masi, Amalia Gomez-Rexrode, and Aingyea Fraser, "Talking about Costs: Innovation in Clinician-Patient Conversations," *Health Affairs Blog*, November 27, 2018, https://www.healthaffairs.org/do/10.1377/hblog20181126.366161/full/.

30. Ibid.

31. Lara Hoffmans, "They Unblinded Me with Science," *Forbes*, March 23, 2012, https://www.forbes.com/sites/larahoffmans/2012/03/23/they-unblinded-me-with-science/#9701c6a216dc.

32. "Healthcare Bluebook," https://www.healthcarebluebook.com/ui/proceduredetails/289?directsearch=true&tab=ShopForCare.

CHAPTER 6

1. Gretchen Herrmann, "Negotiating Culture: Conflict and Consensus in U.S. Garage-Sale Bargaining," *Ethnology* 42, no. 3 (2003): 237–52.

2. Ibid.

3. David Gill and John Thanassoulis, "The Impact of Bargaining on Markets with Price Takers: Too Many Bargainers Spoil the Broth," *European Economic Review* 53, no. 6 (2009): 658–74.

4. Jack O'Brien, "Hospital Bad Debt Rising as Patients Shoulder Bigger Share of Medical Bills," HealthLeaders, June 26, 2018, https://www.healthleadersmedia.com/finance/hospital-bad-debt-rising-patients-shoulder-bigger-share-medical-bills.

5. Barbara Kiviat, "Got Hefty Medical Bills? Try Negotiating to Get Them Reduced," *Consumer Reports*, April 4, 2017, https://www.consumer reports.org/health-insurance/got-hefty-medical-bills-try-negotiating/.

6. Olga Khazan, "Americans Are Going Bankrupt from Getting Sick," *The Atlantic*, March 15, 2019, https://www.theatlantic.com/health/archive/2019/03/hospital-bills-medical-debt-bankruptcy/584998/.

7. Brooke Murphy, "20 Things to Know about Balance Billing," *Becker's Hospital CFO Report*, February 17, 2016, https://www.beckershospitalre view.com/finance/20-things-to-know-about-balance-billing.html.

8. "NHE Fact Sheet: Historical NHE 2017," Centers for Medicare and Medicaid Services, last updated April 26, 2019, https://www.cms.gov/research-statistics-data-and-systems/statistics-trends-and-reports/nationalhealthexpenddata/nhe-fact-sheet.html.

9. Robin A. Cohen, Emily P. Terlizzi, and Michael E. Martinez, "Health Insurance Coverage: Early Release of Estimates from the National Health Interview Survey, 2018," Division of Health Interview Statistics, National Center for Health Statistics, released May 2019, https://www.cdc.gov/nchs/data/nhis/earlyrelease/insur201905.pdf.

10. Lara Sanpietro, "Negotiate the Healthcare Industry," Program on Negotiation, Harvard Law School, *Daily Blog*, December 4, 2018, https://www.pon.harvard.edu/daily/teaching-negotiation-daily/negotiate-the-healthcare-industry/.

11. Preyas Desai and Devavrat Purohit, "'Let Me Talk to My Manager': Haggling in a Competitive Environment," *Marketing Science* 23, no. 2 (2004): 219–33.

12. Susan Jaffe, "No More Secrets: Congress Bans Pharmacist 'Gag Orders' on Drug Prices," *Kaiser Health News*, October 10, 2018, https://khn.org/news/no-more-secrets-congress-bans-pharmacist-gag-orders-on-drug-prices/.

13. Donna Rosato, "What Medical Debt Does to Your Credit Score," *Consumer Reports*, July 26, 2018, https://www.consumerreports.org/credit-scores-reports/what-medical-debt-does-to-your-credit-score/.

CHAPTER 7

1. JaWanna Henry, Wes Barker, and Lolita Kachay, "Electronic Capabilities for Patient Engagement among U.S. Non-Federal Acute Care Hospitals: 2013–2017," The Office of the National Coordinator for Health Information Technology, ONC Data Brief No. 45, April 2019, https://www.healthit.gov/sites/default/files/page/2019-04/AHApatientengagement.pdf.

2. Devesh Raval, "What Determines Customer Complaining Behavior?" Federal Trade Commission, July 30, 2016, https://www.ftc.gov/system/files/documents/public_events/966823/raval_whatdeterminescon sumercomplainingbehavior_0.pdf.

3. Diane Halstead, Michael A. Jones, and April N. Cox, "Satisfaction Theory and the Disadvantaged Consumer," *Journal of Consumer Satisfaction, Dissatisfaction and Complaining Behavior* 20 (2007): 15–35.

4. Dennis E. Garrett and Peter G. Toumanoff, "Are Consumers Disadvantaged or Vulnerable? An Examination of Consumer Complaints to the Better Business Bureau," *Journal of Consumer Affairs* 44, no. 1 (2010): 3–23.

5. "Direct Primary Care Trends Report 2017," cdn2, 2017, https://cdn2 .hubspot.net/hubfs/2562809/pdf-assets/dpc-trends-2017/Hint-DPC-Trends-Report-2017.pdf.

6. Forbes Staff, "'Hi, This Is Sy Sims,'" *Forbes*, November 18, 2009, https://www.forbes.com/2009/11/18/sy-syms-retailer-business-retail-obit uary.html#32e152b54a68.

CHAPTER 8

1. Louis Graff, John Russell, John Seashore, Jan Tate, Ann Elwell, Mark Prete, Mike Werdmann, Rachel Maag, Charles Krivenko, and Martha Radford, "False-Negative and False-Positive Errors in Abdominal Pain Evaluation Failure to Diagnose Acute Appendicitis and Unnecessary Surgery," *Academic Emergency Medicine* 7, no. 11 (2000): 1244–55.

2. Hardeep Singh, Ashley N. D. Meyer, and Eric J. Thomas, "The Frequency of Diagnostic Errors in Outpatient Care: Estimations from Three Large Observational Studies Involving U.S. Adult Populations, "*BMJ Quality & Safety* 23, no. 9 (2014): 727–31.

3. David E. Newman-Toker, Kathryn M. McDonald, David O. Meltzer, G. T. Butchy, H. P. Lehmann, E. M. Aldrich, A. Chanmugam, and K. D. Frick, "How Much Diagnostic Safety Can We Afford, and How Should We Decide? A Health Economics Perspective," *BMJ Quality & Safety* 22, Suppl. 2 (2013): ii11–ii20.

4. Mark L. Graber, "The Incidence of Diagnostic Error in Medicine," *BMJ Quality & Safety* 22, Suppl. 2 (2013): ii21–ii27.

5. Hardeep Singh, Kamal Hirani, Himabindu Kadiyala, Olga Rudomiotov, Traber Davis, Myrna M. Khan, and Terry L. Wahls, "Characteristics and Predictors of Missed Opportunities in Lung Cancer Diagnosis: An Electronic Health Record-Based Study," *Journal of Clinical Oncology: Official Journal of the American Society of Clinical Oncology* 28, no. 20 (2010): 3307–15.

6. Robert M. A. Hirschfeld and Lana A. Vornik, "Recognition and Diagnosis of Bipolar Disorder," *The Journal of Clinical Psychiatry* 65, Suppl. 15 (2004): 5–9.

7. Leana S. Wen and Joshua M. Kosowsky, *When Doctors Don't Listen: How to Avoid Misdiagnoses and Unnecessary Tests*, first edition (New York: Thomas Dunne Books, St. Martin's Press, 2013).

8. Esther H. Chen, Frances S. Shofer, Anthony J. Dean, Judd E. Hollander, William G. Baxt, Jennifer L. Robey, Keara L. Sease, and Angela M. Mills, "Gender Disparity in Analgesic Treatment of Emergency Department Patients with Acute Abdominal Pain," *Academic Emergency Medicine* 15, no. 5 (2008): 414–18.

9. E. J. Bartley, R. B. Fillingim, L. Colvin, and D. J. Rowbotham, "Sex Differences in Pain: A Brief Review of Clinical and Experimental Findings," *British Journal of Anaesthesia* 111, no. 1 (2013): 52–58.

10. Roger Fillingim, Christopher King, Margarete Ribeiro-Dasilva, Bridgett Rahim-Williams, and Joseph Riley, "Sex, Gender, and Pain: A Review of Recent Clinical and Experimental Findings," *Journal of Pain* 10, no. 5 (2009): 447–85.

11. David Ruau, Linda Liu, David Clark, Martin Angst, and Atul Butte, "Sex Differences in Reported Pain across 11,000 Patients Captured in Electronic Medical Records," *Journal of Pain* 13, no. 3 (2012): 228–34.

12. Karen Calderone, "The Influence of Gender on the Frequency of Pain and Sedative Medication Administered to Postoperative Patients," *Sex Roles: A Journal of Research* 23, no. 11–12 (1990): 713–25.

13. Heather Ashton, "Psychotropic-Drug Prescribing for Women," *British Journal of Psychiatry* 158, no. S10 (1991): 30–35.

14. Siobhan Fenton, "How Sexist Stereotypes Mean Doctors Ignore Women's Pain," *Independent*, July 27, 2016, https://www.independent.co.uk/life-style/health-and-families/health-news/how-sexist-stereotypes-mean-doctors-ignore-womens-pain-a7157931.html.

15. Joe Fassler, "How Doctors Take Women's Pain Less Seriously," *The Atlantic*, October 15, 2015, https://www.theatlantic.com/health/archive/2015/10/emergency-room-wait-times-sexism/410515/.

16. Jazmine Joyner, "Nobody Believes That Black Women Are in Pain and It's Killing Us," WearYourVoicemag.com, May 25, 2018, https://wearyourvoicemag.com/race/black-women-are-in-pain.

17. Kate Beaton, "Our Sister Becky: What If the Doctors Had Listened to Her?" The Cut, September 20, 2018, https://www.thecut.com/2018/09/what-if-the-doctors-had-listened-to-our-sister-becky.html?fbclid=IwAR3zHQaetOlX0D55ndERNsYFG675G1LahN2repa1e-PD2XdVZ5mpa2oo7bw.

18. J. Hector Pope, Tom P. Aufderheide, Robin Ruthazer, Robert H. Woolard, James A. Feldman, Joni R. Beshansky, John L. Griffith, and Harry P. Selker, "Missed Diagnoses of Acute Cardiac Ischemia in the Emergency Department," *The New England Journal of Medicine* 342, no. 16 (2000): 1163–70.

19. Matt Simon, "Fantastically Wrong: The Theory of the Wandering Wombs That Drove Women to Madness," *Wired*, May 7, 2014, https://www.wired.com/2014/05/fantastically-wrong-wandering-womb/.

20. Harold Merskey and Paul Potter, "The Womb Lay Still in Ancient Egypt," *British Journal of Psychiatry* 154, no. 6 (1989): 751–53.

21. Catherine Pearson, "Female Hysteria: 7 Crazy Things People Used to Believe about the Ladies' Disease," *HuffPost*, November 21, 2013, https://www.huffpost.com/entry/female-hysteria_n_4298060.

22. Guy David, Candace Gunnarsson, Heidi Waters, Ruslan Horblyuk, and Harold Kaplan, "Economic Measurement of Medical Errors Using a Hospital Claims Database," *Value in Health* 16, no. 2 (2012): 305–10.

23. Jill Van Den Bos, Karan Rustagi, Travis Gray, Michael Halford, Eva Ziemkiewicz, and Jonathan Shreve, "The $17.1 Billion Problem: The Annual Cost of Measurable Medical Errors," *Health Affairs* 30, no. 4 (2011): 596–603.

24. Jon Shreve, Jill Van Den Bos, Travis Gray, Michael Halford, Karan Rustagi, and Eva Ziemkiewicz, "The Economic Measurement of Medical Errors," Society of Actuaries' Health Section, Milliman, June 2010, https://www.soa.org/globalassets/assets/files/research/projects/research-econ-measurement.pdf.

25. Martin A. Makary and Michael Daniel, "Medical Error—The Third Leading Cause of Death in the U.S.," *BMJ* 353 (2016): I2139.

26. "Robert Veatch, PhD," The Kennedy Institute of Ethics, https://kennedyinstitute.georgetown.edu/people/robert-veatch/.

27. Anne M. Stiggelbout, Arwen H. Pieterse, and Johanna C. De Haes, "Shared Decision Making: Concepts, Evidence, and Practice," *Patient Education and Counseling* 98, no. 10 (2015): 1172–79.

28. Chad Cook, "Is Clinical Gestalt Good Enough?" *Journal of Manual & Manipulative Therapy* 17, no. 1 (2009): 6–7.

29. Pat Croskerry, "The Importance of Cognitive Errors in Diagnosis and Strategies to Minimize Them," *Academic Medicine* 78, no. 8 (2003): 775–80.

30. Eta S. Berner and Mark L. Graber, "Overconfidence as a Cause of Diagnostic Error in Medicine," *The American Journal of Medicine* 121, no. 5 (2008): S2–S23.

31. David L. Schriger, Joshua W. Elder, and Richelle J. Cooper, "Structured Clinical Decision Aids Are Seldom Compared with Subjective Physician Judgment, and Are Seldom Superior," *Annals of Emergency Medicine* 70, no. 3 (2017): 338–44.e3.

32. John E. Wennberg, "Dealing with Medical Practice Variations: A Proposal for Action," *Health Affairs* 3, no. 2 (1984): 6–32.

33. Stiggelbout, Pieterse, and De Haes, "Shared Decision Making."

34. Ibid.

35. David Veroff, Amy Marr, and David E. Wennberg, "Enhanced Support for Shared Decision Making Reduced Costs of Care for Patients with Preference-Sensitive Conditions," *Health Affairs* 32, no. 2 (2013): 285–93.

36. David Arterburn, Robert Wellman, Emily Westbrook, Carolyn Rutter, Tyler Ross, David Mcculloch, Matthew Handley, and Charles Jung, "Introducing Decision Aids at Group Health Was Linked to Sharply Lower Hip and Knee Surgery Rates and Costs," *Health Affairs* 31, no. 9 (2012): 2094–104.

37. Emily Oshima Lee and Ezekiel J. Emanuel, "Shared Decision Making to Improve Care and Reduce Costs," *The New England Journal of Medicine* 368, no. 1 (2013): 6–8.

38. Ibid.

39. Ming Tai-Seale, Thomas G. McGuire, and Weimin Zhang, "Time Allocation in Primary Care Office Visits," *Health Services Research* 42, no. 5 (2007): 1871–94.

40. Sarah Grisham, "Medscape Physician Compensation Report 2017," Medscape, April 5, 2017, https://www.medscape.com/slideshow/compensation-2017-overview-6008547#33.

41. Sonia Bernardes, Margarida Costa, and Helena Carvalho, "Engendering Pain Management Practices: The Role of Physician Sex on Chronic Low-Back Pain Assessment and Treatment Prescriptions," *Journal of Pain* 14, no. 9 (2013): 931–40.

42. Brad Greenwood, Seth Carnahan, and Laura Huang, "Patient-Physician Gender Concordance and Increased Mortality among Female Heart Attack Patients," *Proceedings of the National Academy of Sciences of the United States of America* 115, no. 34 (2018): 8569–74.

43. Yusuke Tsugawa, Anupam B. Jena, Jose F. Figueroa, E. John Orav, Daniel M. Blumenthal, and Ashish K. Jha, "Comparison of Hospital Mortality and Readmission Rates for Medicare Patients Treated by Male vs. Female Physicians," *JAMA Internal Medicine* 177, no. 2 (2017): 206–13.

44. Greenwood, Carnahan, and Huang, "Patient-Physician Gender Concordance."

CHAPTER 9

1. "Richard Branson, Quotes, Quotable Quotes," Goodreads, https://www.goodreads.com/quotes/7356284-clients-do-not-come-first-employees-come-first-if-you.

2. "Understanding Quality Measurement," Agency for Healthcare Research and Quality, last updated October 2018, https://www.ahrq.gov/professionals/quality-patient-safety/quality-resources/tools/chtoolbx/understand/index.html.

3. "Finding Quality Doctors: How Americans Evaluate Provider Quality in the United States," Associated Press-NORC Center for Public Affairs Research, July 2014, http://www.apnorc.org/PDFs/Finding%20Quality%20Doctors/Finding%20Quality%20Doctors%20Research%20Highlights.pdf.

4. "HEDIS Measures and Technical Resources," National Committee for Quality Assurance, https://www.ncqa.org/hedis/measures/.

5. "Adult BMI Assessment (ABA)," National Committee for Quality Assurance, https://www.ncqa.org/hedis/measures/adult-bmi-assessment/.

6. Will Koehrsen, "Unintended Consequences and Goodhart's Law," Towards Data Science, February 24, 2018, https://towardsdatascience .com/unintended-consequences-and-goodharts-law-68d60a94705c.

7. "Finding Quality Doctors."

8. Ibid.

9. Ibid.

10. Ibid.

11. Bruce A. Arnow, Dana Steidtmann, Christine Blasey, Rachel Manber, Michael J. Constantino, Daniel N. Klein, John C. Markowitz, Barbara O. Rothbaum, Michael E. Thase, Aaron J. Fisher, and James H. Kocsis, "The Relationship between the Therapeutic Alliance and Treatment Outcome in Two Distinct Psychotherapies for Chronic Depression," *Journal of Consulting and Clinical Psychology* 81, no. 4 (2013): 627–38.

12. Elizabeth Murray, Lance Pollack, Martha White, and Bernard Lo, "Clinical Decision-Making: Physicians' Preferences and Experiences," *BMC Family Practice* 8 (2007): 10.

13. Kristin Carman, Maureen Maurer, Jill Yegian, Pamela Dardess, Jeanne McGee, Mark Evers, and Karen Marlo, "Evidence That Consumers Are Skeptical about Evidence-Based Health Care," *Health Affairs* 29, no. 7 (2010): 1400–06.

14. Atul Gawande, *The Checklist Manifesto: How to Get Things Right*, first edition (New York: Metropolitan Books, 2010).

15. Carman, Maurer, Yegian, Dardess, McGee, Evers, and Marlo, "Evidence That Consumers Are Skeptical about Evidence-Based Health Care."

16. Nate Silver, *The Signal and the Noise: Why So Many Predictions Fail—But Some Don't* (New York: Penguin Press, 2012).

17. "Finding Quality Doctors."

CHAPTER 10

1. "List of Medicaid Eligibility Groups," Medicaid.gov, https://www .medicaid.gov/medicaid-chip-program-information/by-topics/waivers/ 1115/downloads/list-of-eligibility-groups.pdf.

2. Deborah Gordon, "How Many Businesses Won't Start If ObamaCare Is Repealed?" TheHill.com, March 1, 2017, https://thehill.com/blogs/pundits-blog/economy-budget/321761-how-many-businesses-wont-start-if-obamacare-is-repealed.

3. U.S. Small Business Administration, *2018 Small Business Profile* (Washington, DC: U.S. Small Business Administration, Office of Advocacy,

2018), https://www.sba.gov/sites/default/files/advocacy/2018-Small-Business-Profiles-US.pdf.

4. Ibid.

5. Dean Baker, "Job Lock and Employer-Provided Health Insurance: Evidence from the Literature," Research Report (Center for Economic and Policy Research, AARP Public Policy Institute, March 2015).

6. Robert W. Fairlie, Kanika Kapur, and Susan Gates, "Is Employer-Based Health Insurance a Barrier to Entrepreneurship?" *Journal of Health Economics* 30, no. 1 (2011): 146–62.

7. Baker, "Job Lock and Employer-Provided Health Insurance."

8. Steven Nyce, Sylvester J. Schieber, John B. Shoven, Sita Nataraj Slavov, and David A. Wise, "Does Retiree Health Insurance Encourage Early Retirement?" *Journal of Public Economics* 104 (2013): 40–51.

9. Inas Rashad and Eric Sarpong, "Employer-Provided Health Insurance and the Incidence of Job Lock: A Literature Review and Empirical Test," *Expert Review of Pharmacoeconomics & Outcomes Research* 8, no. 6 (12, 2008): 583–91.

10. Baker, "Job Lock and Employer-Provided Health Insurance."

11. Daniel Sgroi, "Happiness and Productivity: Understanding the Happy-Productive Worker," *Social Market Foundation Global Perspectives Series*, Paper 4, October 2015, http://www.smf.co.uk/wp-content/uploads/2015/10/Social-Market-Foundation-Publication-Briefing-CAGE-4-Are-happy-workers-more-productive-281015.pdf#page=9.

12. Johanna Stengård, Claudia Bernhard-Oettel, Erik Berntson, Constanze Leineweber, and Gunnar Aronsson, "Stuck in a Job: Being 'Locked-In' or at Risk of Becoming Locked-In at the Workplace and Well-Being over Time," *Work and Stress* 30, no. 2 (2016): 152–72.

13. Edward R. Berchick, Emily Hood, and Jessica C. Barnett, *Health Insurance Coverage in the United States: 2017* (Washington, DC: United States Census Bureau, September 2018), https://www.census.gov/library/publications/2018/demo/p60-264.html.

14. United States Bureau of the Census, "Vital Statistics and Health and Medical Care," *Historical Statistics of the United States: Colonial Times to 1970—Part 1* (Washington, DC: U.S. Department of Commerce, Bureau of the Census, 1975), https://www2.census.gov/prod2/statcomp/documents/CT1970p1-03.pdf.

15. Harold T. Shapiro, Marilyn J. Field, Institute of Medicine, and Committee on Employment-Based Health Benefits, "Employment and Health Benefits: A Connection at Risk" (Washington, DC: National Academies Press, 2000).

16. J. E. Affeldt, "Voluntary Accreditation," *Proceedings of the Academy of Political Science* 33, no. 4 (1980): 182–91.

17. George B. Moseley, "The U.S. Health Care Non-System, 1908–2008," *The Virtual Mentor: VM* 10, no. 5 (2008): 324–31.

18. Ibid.

19. Shapiro and Field, "Employment and Health Benefits."

20. Stephen Mihm, "Employer-Based Health Care Was a Wartime Accident," *Chicago Tribune*, February 24, 2017, https://www.chicagotri bune.com/opinion/commentary/ct-obamacare-health-care-employers-20170224-story.html.

21. History.com Editors, "American Women in World War II," *History .com*, August 21, 2018, https://www.history.com/topics/world-war-ii/american-women-in-world-war-ii-1.

22. Mihm, "Employer-Based Health Care Was a Wartime Accident."

23. Sean Gorman, "Carr Says Few People Had Health Insurance Prior to World War II," *Politifact.com*, October 30, 2014, https://www.politifact .com/virginia/statements/2014/oct/30/james-carr/carr-says-prior-wwii-very-few-people-had-health-in/;.

24. Robin A. Cohen, Diane M. Makuc, Amy B. Bernstein, Linda T. Bilheimer, and Eve Powell-Griner, "Health Insurance Coverage Trends, 1959–2007: Estimates from the National Health Interview Survey" (Hyattsville, MD: National Center for Health Statistics, 2009), https://www.cdc .gov/nchs/data/nhsr/nhsr017.pdf.

25. United States Bureau of the Census, "Vital Statistics," https://www2.census.gov/prod2/statcomp/documents/CT1970p1-03.pdf.

26. Trent Burner, Liz Supinksi, Susan Zhu, Samuel Robinson, and Cate Supinski, "The Global Skills Shortage: Bridging the Talent Gap with Education, Training and Sourcing" (Society for Human Resources Management, 2019), https://www.shrm.org/hr-today/trends-and-forecasting/research-and-surveys/Documents/SHRM%20Skills%20Gap%202019 .pdf.

27. "The Gig Economy and Alternative Work Arrangements," Gallup, 2018, https://www.gallup.com/workplace/240878/gig-economy-paper-2018 .aspx.

28. Diane Mulcahy, *The Gig Economy: The Complete Guide to Getting Better Work, Taking More Time Off, and Financing the Life You Want*, first edition (New York, NY: AMACOM, 2016).

29. Lynn A. Karoly and Constantijn (Stan) Panis, "The Future at Work: Trends and Implications," Research Brief RB-5070-DOL (Rand Corporation, 2004), https://www.rand.org/pubs/research_briefs/RB5070.html.

30. Stephen Miller, "6 Big Benefits Trends for 2019," Society for Human Resources Management, January 3, 2019, https://www.shrm.org/resource sandtools/hr-topics/benefits/pages/big-benefit-trends-2019.aspx.

31. Gary Claxton, Matthew Rae, Michelle Long, Anthony Damico, Gregory Young, Daniel McDermott, and Heidi Whitmore, "Employer Health Benefits 2019 Annual Survey," Kaiser Family Foundation, 2019, http://files.kff.org/attachment/Report-Employer-Health-Benefits-Annual-Survey-2019.

32. Sara R. Collins and David C. Radley, "The Cost of Employer Insurance Is a Growing Burden for Middle-Income Families," Data Brief, The Commonwealth Fund, December 2018, https://www.commonwealthfund.org/sites/default/files/2018-12/Collins_state_premium_trends_2018_db_0.pdf.

33. Regina E. Herzlinger, Barak D. Richman, and Richard J. Boxer, "How Health Care Hurts Your Paycheck," *The New York Times*, November 2, 2016, https://www.nytimes.com/2016/11/02/opinion/how-health-care-hurts-your-paycheck.html.

34. Herzlinger, Richman, and Boxer, "How Health Care Hurts Your Paycheck."

35. Claxton, Rae, Long, Damico, Young, McDermott, and Whitmore, "Employer Health Benefits 2019 Annual Survey."

36. Collins and Radley, "The Cost of Employer Insurance."

37. Liz Hamel, Cailey Muñana, and Mollyann Brodie, "Kaiser Family Foundation/LA Times Survey of Adults with Employer-Sponsored Insurance," Kaiser Family Foundation, May 2, 2019, https://www.kff.org/report-section/kaiser-family-foundation-la-times-survey-of-adults-with-employer-sponsored-insurance-section-1-profile-of-adults-with-employer-sponsored-health-insurance-and-overall-views-of-coverage/.

38. Ibid.

39. Kathleen Elkins, "Here's How Much Money Americans Have in Savings at Every Income Level," CNBC Make It, September 27, 2018, https://www.cnbc.com/2018/09/27/heres-how-much-money-americans-have-in-savings-at-every-income-level.html.

40. Cameron Huddleston, "58% of Americans Have Less than $1,000 in Savings," GoBankingRates, May 24, 2019, https://www.gobankingrates.com/saving-money/savings-advice/58-of-americans-have-less-than-1000-in-savings/.

41. Anna Bahney, "40% of Americans Can't Cover a $400 Emergency Expense," *CNN Money*, May 22, 2018, https://money.cnn.com/2018/05/22/pf/emergency-expenses-household-finances/index.html.

42. Noam N. Levey, "Health Insurance Deductibles Soar, Leaving Americans with Unaffordable Bills," *Los Angeles Times*, May 2, 2019, https://www.latimes.com/politics/la-na-pol-health-insurance-medical-bills-20190502-story.html.

43. Hamel, Muñana, and Brodie, "Kaiser Family Foundation/LA Times Survey."

44. Levey, "Health Insurance Deductibles Soar."

45. Ibid.

46. Sara R. Collins, Herman K. Bhupal, and Michelle M. Doty, "Health Insurance Coverage Eight Years after the ACA," The Commonwealth Fund, February 7, 2019, https://www.commonwealthfund.org/publications/issue-briefs/2019/feb/health-insurance-coverage-eight-years-after-aca.

47. Aaron Carroll, "The Real Reason the U.S. Has Employer-Sponsored Health Insurance," *The New York Times*, September 5, 2017, https://www.nytimes.com/2017/09/05/upshot/the-real-reason-the-us-has-employer-sponsored-health-insurance.html.

48. Herzlinger, Richman, Boxer, "How Health Care Hurts Your Paycheck."

49. Bruce Bartlett, "The Question of Taxing Employer-Provided Health Insurance," *The New York Times Economix*, July 30, 2013, https://economix.blogs.nytimes.com/2013/07/30/the-question-of-taxing-employer-provided-health-insurance.

50. Ibid.

51. Ibid.

CHAPTER 11

1. Sara R. Collins, Herman K. Bhupal, and Michelle M. Doty, "Health Insurance Coverage Eight Years after the ACA," The Commonwealth Fund, February 7, 2019, https://www.commonwealthfund.org/publications/issue-briefs/2019/feb/health-insurance-coverage-eight-years-after-aca.

2. Rachel Fehr, Cynthia Cox, and Larry Levitt, "Data Note: Changes in Enrollment in the Individual Health Insurance Market through Early 2019," Kaiser Family Foundation, August 21, 2019, https://www.kff.org/private-insurance/issue-brief/data-note-changes-in-enrollment-in-the-individual-health-insurance-market-through-early-2019/.

3. "4 Basic Health Insurance Terms 96% of Americans Don't Understand," Policy Genius, January 24, 2018, https://www.policygenius.com/health-insurance/learn/health-insurance-literacy-survey/.

4. Alicia L. Nobles, Brett A. Curtis, Duc A. Ngo, Emily Vardell, and Christopher P. Holstege, "Health Insurance Literacy: A Mixed Methods Study of College Students," *Journal of American College Health* 67, no. 5 (2018): 1–10.

5. "The Hidden Cost of Healthcare System Complexity," Accenture, 2018, https://www.accenture.com/_acnmedia/pdf-104/accenture-health-hidden-cost-of-healthcare-system-complexity.pdf.

6. Ibid.

7. Saurabh Bhargava, George Loewenstein, and Justin Sydnor, "Do Individuals Make Sensible Health Insurance Decisions? Evidence from a Menu with Dominated Options," *NBER Working Paper Series*, 2015, 21160.

8. Ibid.

9. "The Hidden Cost."

10. Renuka Tipirneni, Mary C. Politi, Jeffrey T. Kullgren, Edith C. Kieffer, Susan D. Goold, and Aaron M. Scherer, "Association between Health

Insurance Literacy and Avoidance of Health Care Services Owing to Cost," *JAMA Network Open* 1, no. 7 (2018): E184796.

11. Sharon K. Long and Dana Goin, "Large Racial and Ethnic Differences in Health Insurance Literacy Signal Need for Targeted Education and Outreach," Health Reform Monitoring Survey, Urban Institute Health Policy Center, February 6, 2014, http://hrms.urban.org/briefs/literacy-by-race.html.

12. "Talking about Jargon," Healthliteracy.com, April 9, 2013, https://healthliteracy.com/2013/04/09/talking-about-jargon-hlol-94/.

13. Nobles, Curtis, Ngo, Vardell, and Holstege, "Health Insurance Literacy."

14. Economic News Release, "Employer Costs for Employee Compensation," Bureau of Labor Statistics, June 18, 2019, https://www.bls.gov/news.release/ecec.nr0.htm.

15. Christopher S. Girod, Susan K. Hart, David M. Liner, Thomas D. Snook, and Scott A. Weltz, "2019 Milliman Medical Index," July 25, 2019, http://www.milliman.com/mmi/.

16. https://www.healthcare.gov/glossary/co-payment/.

17. https://www.healthcare.gov/glossary/premium/.

18. Gary Claxton, Larry Levitt, Michelle Long, and Erik Blumenkranz, "Increases in Cost-Sharing Payments Have Far Outpaced Wage Growth," Peterson-Kaiser Health System Tracker, October 4, 2017, https://www.healthsystemtracker.org/brief/increases-in-cost-sharing-payments-have-far-outpaced-wage-growth/.

19. "How Do Deductibles, Coinsurance and Copays Work?" Blue Cross Blue Shield, https://www.bcbsm.com/index/health-insurance-help/faqs/topics/how-health-insurance-works/deductibles-coinsurance-copays.html.

20. Nobles, Curtis, Ngo, Vardell, and Holstege, "Health Insurance Literacy."

21. https://www.healthcare.gov/glossary/deductible/.

22. https://www.healthcare.gov/glossary/out-of-pocket-maximum-limit/.

23. https://www.healthcare.gov/glossary/formulary/.

24. https://www.healthcare.gov/glossary/annual-limit/.

25. https://www.healthcare.gov/glossary/prior-authorization/.

26. https://www.healthcare.gov/glossary/health-maintenance-organization-hmo/.

27. https://www.healthcare.gov/glossary/health-reimbursement-account-hra/.

28. https://www.healthcare.gov/glossary/health-savings-account-hsa/.

29. https://www.healthcare.gov/glossary/flexible-spending-account-fsa/.

CHAPTER 12

1. William Samuelson and Richard Zeckhauser, "Status Quo Bias in Decision Making," *Journal of Risk and Uncertainty* 1, no. 1 (1988): 7–59.

2. Saurabh Bhargava, George Loewenstein, and Justin Sydnor, "Do Individuals Make Sensible Health Insurance Decisions? Evidence from a Menu with Dominated Options," *NBER Working Paper Series*, 2015, 21160.

3. David M. Cutler and Richard Zeckhauser, "Extending the Theory to Meet the Practice of Insurance," *Brookings-Wharton Papers on Financial Services* 2004 (2004): 1–53.

4. Richard Frank and Karine Lamiraud, "Choice, Price Competition and Complexity in Markets for Health Insurance," *Journal of Economic Behavior and Organization* 71, no. 2 (2009): 550–62.

5. Regina E. Herzlinger, *Who Killed Health Care? America's $2 Trillion Medical Problem—and the Consumer-Driven Cure* (New York: McGraw Hill, 2007).

CHAPTER 13

1. Gary Claxton, Larry Levitt, and Michelle Long, "Payments for Cost Sharing Increasing Rapidly over Time," Peterson-Kaiser Health System Tracker, April 12, 2016, https://www.healthsystemtracker.org/brief/payments-for-cost-sharing-increasing-rapidly-over-time/#item-start.

2. Gary Claxton, Larry Levitt, Michelle Long, and Erik Blumenkranz, "Increases in Cost-Sharing Payments Have Far Outpaced Wage Growth," Peterson-Kaiser Health System Tracker, October 4, 2017, https://www.healthsystemtracker.org/brief/increases-in-cost-sharing-payments-have-far-outpaced-wage-growth/.

3. Centers for Medicare and Medicaid Services (CMS). NHE Fact Sheet, Centers for Medicare and Medicaid Services, April 17, 2018, https://www.cms.gov/research-statistics-data-and-systems/statistics-trends-and-reports/nationalhealthexpenddata/nhe-fact-sheet.html.

4. Rand Health, "Determining the Effects of Cost-Sharing in Health Care," Rand Corporation, https://www.rand.org/capabilities/solutions/determining-the-effects-of-cost-sharing-in-health-care.html.

5. Melinda Beeuwkes Buntin, Cheryl Damberg, Amelia Haviland, Kanika Kapur, Nicole Lurie, Roland McDevitt, and M. Susan Marquis, "Consumer-Directed Health Care: Early Evidence about Effects on Cost and Quality," *Health Affairs* 25, no. 6 (2006): W516–30.

6. Joseph P. Newhouse, "Consumer-Directed Health Plans and the RAND Health Insurance Experiment," *Health Affairs* 23, no. 6 (2004): 107–13.

7. Zarek C. Brot-Goldberg, Amitabh Chandra, Benjamin R. Handel, and Jonathan T. Kolstad, "What Does a Deductible Do? The Impact of Cost-Sharing on Health Care Prices, Quantities, and Spending Dynamics," *The Quarterly Journal of Economics* 132, no. 3 (2017): 1261–318.

8. Rajender Agarwal, Olena Mazurenko, and Nir Menachemi, "High-Deductible Health Plans Reduce Health Care Cost and Utilization, Including Use of Needed Preventive Services," *Health Affairs* 36, no. 10 (2017): 1762–1768.

9. J. Frank Wharam, Fang Zhang, Jamie Wallace, Christine Lu, Craig Earle, Stephen B. Soumerai, Larissa Nekhlyudov, and Dennis Ross-Degnan, "Vulnerable and Less Vulnerable Women in High-Deductible Health Plans Experienced Delayed Breast Cancer Care," *Health Affairs* 38, no. 3 (2019): 408–15.

10. J. Frank Wharam, Fang Zhang, Emma M. Eggleston, Christine Y. Lu, Stephen B. Soumerai, and Dennis Ross-Degnan, "Effect of High-Deductible Insurance on High-Acuity Outcomes in Diabetes: A Natural Experiment for Translation in Diabetes (NEXT-D) Study," *Diabetes Care* 41, no. 5 (2018): 940–48.

11. Beatrix Hoffman, "Restraining the Health Care Consumer: The History of Deductibles and Co-payments in U.S. Health Insurance," *Social Science History* 30, no. 4 (2006): 501–528.

12. Joseph P. Newhouse and Rand Corporation, Insurance Experiment Group, *Free for All? Lessons from the Rand Health Insurance Experiment: A RAND Study* (Cambridge, MA: Harvard University Press, 1993).

13. Joseph P. Newhouse, "A Summary of the Rand Health Insurance Study," *Annals of the New York Academy of Sciences* 387 (1982): 111–14.

14. Newhouse, "Consumer-Directed Health Plans."

15. Hoffman, "Restraining the Health Care Consumer."

16. Robert H. Brook, Emmett B. Keeler, Kathleen N. Lohr, Joseph P. Newhouse, John E. Ware, William H. Rogers, Allyson Ross Davies, Cathy D. Sherbourne, George A. Goldberg, Patricia Camp, Caren Kamberg, Arleen Leibowitz, Joan Keesey, and David Reboussin, "The Health Insurance Experiment: A Classic RAND Study Speaks to the Current Health Care Reform Debate" (Santa Monica, CA: RAND Corporation, 2006), https://www.rand.org/pubs/research_briefs/RB9174.htmlhttps://www.rand.org/pubs/research_briefs/RB9174.html.

17. Gary Claxton, Matthew Rae, Michelle Long, Anthony Damico, Gregory Young, Daniel McDermott, and Heidi Whitmore, "Employer Health Benefits 2019 Annual Survey," Kaiser Family Foundation, 2019, http://files.kff.org/attachment/Report-Employer-Health-Benefits-Annual-Survey-2019.

18. Sara R. Collins and David C. Radley, "The Cost of Employer Insurance Is a Growing Burden for Middle-Income Families," Data Brief, The Commonwealth Fund, December 2018, https://www.commonwealthfund.org/sites/default/files/2018-12/Collins_state_premium_trends_2018_db_0.pdf.

19. Claxton, Rae, Long, Damico, Young, McDermott, and Whitmore, "Employer Health Benefits 2019 Annual Survey."

20. "Average Health Care Deductible Nearly $1,500 for Individual Coverage through an Employer Plan," International Foundation of Employee

Health Benefits, last modified September 11, 2018, https://www.ifebp.org/aboutus/pressroom/releases/Pages/Average-Health-Care-Deductible-Nearly-$1,500-for-Individual-Coverage-Through-an-Employer-Plan.aspx.

21. Claxton, Rae, Long, Damico, Young, McDermott, and Whitmore, "Employer Health Benefits 2019 Annual Survey."

22. Ibid.

23. Ibid.

24. Ibid.

25. Ibid.

26. Matthew Rae, Rebecca Copeland, and Cynthia Cox, *Tracking the Rise in Premium Contributions and Cost-Sharing for Families with Large Employer Coverage* (Washington, DC: Kaiser Family Foundation, August 14, 2019), https://healthsystemtracker.org/brief/tracking-the-rise-in-premium-contributions-and-cost-sharing-for-families-with-large-employer-coverage.

27. Diana Farrell and Fiona Greig, "Paying Out-of-Pocket: The Healthcare Spending of 2 Million U.S. Families," JP Morgan Chase Institute, September 2009, https://www.jpmorganchase.com/content/dam/jpmorganchase/en/legacy/corporate/institute/document/institute-healthcare.pdf.

28. Martin B. Hackman, Jonathan T. Kolstad, and Amanda E. Kowalski, "Adverse Selection and an Individual Mandate: When Theory Meets Practice," *American Economic Review* 105, no. 3 (2015): 1030–66, https://pubs.aeaweb.org/doi/pdfplus/10.1257/aer.20130758.

29. "Federal Subsidies for Health Insurance Coverage for People under Age 65: 2018 to 2028," Congressional Budget Office, May 2018, https://www.cbo.gov/system/files/115th-congress-2017-2018/reports/53826-healthinsurancecoverage.pdf.

30. Christine Eibner and Sarah Nowak, "The Effect of Eliminating the Individual Mandate Penalty and the Role of Behavioral Factors," The Commonwealth Fund, last modified July 11, 2018, https://www.commonwealthfund.org/publications/fund-reports/2018/jul/eliminating-individual-mandate-penalty-behavioral-factors.

31. Rachel Fehr, Cynthia Cox, and Larry Levitt, "Data Note: Changes in Enrollment in the Individual Health Insurance Market through Early 2019," Kaiser Family Foundation, August 21, 2019, https://www.kff.org/private-insurance/issue-brief/data-note-changes-in-enrollment-in-the-individual-health-insurance-market-through-early-2019/.

32. Noam N. Levey, "Health Insurance Deductibles Soar, Leaving Americans with Unaffordable Bills," *Los Angeles Times*, May 2, 2019, https://www.latimes.com/politics/la-na-pol-health-insurance-medical-bills-20190502-story.html.

33. Liz Hamel, Mira Norton, Karnen Pollitz, Larry Levitt, Gary Claxton, and Mollyann Brodie, "The Burden of Medical Debt: Results from the Kaiser Family Foundation/*New York Times* Medical Bills Survey,"

Henry J Kaiser Family Foundation, last modified January 5, 2016, https://www.kff.org/report-section/the-burden-of-medical-debt-section-3-consequences-of-medical-bill-problems/.

34. David U. Himmelstein, Robert M. Lawless, Deborah Thorne, Pamela Foohey, and Steffie Woolhandler, "Medical Bankruptcy: Still Common Despite the Affordable Care Act," *American Journal of Public Health* 109, no. 3 (2019): 431–433.

35. Rachel Bluth, "GoFundMe CEO: 'Gigantic Gaps' in Health System Showing Up in Crowdfunding," *Kaiser Health News*, January 16, 2019, https://khn.org/news/gofundme-ceo-gigantic-gaps-in-health-system-showing-up-in-crowdfunding/.

36. "Patients May Be the New Payers, But Two in Three Do Not Pay Their Hospital Bills in Full," TransUnion, last modified June 26, 2017, https://newsroom.transunion.com/patients-may-be-the-new-payers-but-two-in-three-do-not-pay-their-hospital-bills-in-full/.

37. "Key Facts about the Uninsured Population," Kaiser Family Foundation, December 7, 2018, https://www.kff.org/uninsured/fact-sheet/key-facts-about-the-uninsured-population/.

38. Rachel Fehr, Cynthia Cox, and Larry Levitt, "Insurer Participation on ACA Marketplaces, 2014–2019," Kaiser Family Foundation, November 14, 2018, https://www.kff.org/health-reform/issue-brief/insurer-participation-on-aca-marketplaces-2014-2019/

39. Mark Vallet, "A Guide to Understanding Your Health Insurance Policy," Insure.com, last modified October 17, 2017, https://www.insure.com/health-insurance/understanding-health-insurance.html.

40. Elisabeth Rosenthal, *An American Sickness: How Healthcare Became Big Business and How You Can Take It Back* (New York: Penguin Press, 2017).

CHAPTER 14

1. Mary Otto, *Teeth: The Story of Beauty, Inequality, and the Struggle for Oral Health in America* (New York: New Press, 2016).

2. Ibid., p. 97.

3. Ibid., p. 105.

4. Lisa Simon, "Overcoming Historical Separation between Oral and General Health Care: Interprofessional Collaboration for Promoting Health Equity," *AMA Journal of Ethics*, September 2016, 18, no. 9 (2016): 941–49.

5. Britt C. Reid, Joan L. Warren, and Gary Rozier, "Comorbidity and Early Diagnosis of Head and Neck Cancer in a Medicare Population," *American Journal of Preventive Medicine* 27, no. 5 (2004): 373–78.

6. Astha Singhal, Elizabeth T. Momany, Michael P. Jones, Daniel J. Caplan, Raymond A. Kuthy, Christopher T. Buresh, and Peter C. Damiano, "Dental Care after an Emergency Department Visit for Dental Problems among Adults Enrolled in Medicaid," *The Journal of the American Dental Association* 147, no. 2 (2016): 111–19.

7. Sara R. Collins, Munira Z. Gunja, Michelle, M. Dotty, and Herman K. Bhupal, "First Look at Health Insurance Coverage in 2018 Finds ACA Gains Beginning to Reverse," The Commonwealth Fund, May 18, 2018, https://www.commonwealthfund.org/blog/2018/first-look-health-insurance-coverage-2018-finds-aca-gains-beginning-reverse.

8. Kamyar Nasseh and Marko Vujicic, "Dental Benefits Coverage Rates Increased for Children and Young Adults in 2013," *Research Brief* (Health Policy Institute, American Dental Association, October 2015).

9. U.S. Dental Expenditures, 2017 Update (Health Policy Institute, American Dental Association, 2017).

10. Marko Vujicic, Thomas Buchmueller, and Rachel Klein, "Dental Care Presents the Highest Level of Financial Barriers, Compared to Other Types of Health Care Services," *Health Affairs* 35, no. 12 (2016): 2176–82.

11. Elizabeth Hinton and Julia Paradise, "Access to Dental Care in Medicaid: Spotlight on Nonelderly Adults," Kaiser Family Foundation, March 17, 2016, https://www.kff.org/medicaid/issue-brief/access-to-dental-care-in-medicaid-spotlight-on-nonelderly-adults/.

12. Sarah Kliff, "One in Three Americans Didn't See the Dentist Last Year," Vox.com, May 4, 2014, https://www.vox.com/2014/5/4/5675878/one-in-three-americans-didnt-see-the-dentist-last-year.

13. Ferris Jabr, "The Trouble with Dentistry," *The Atlantic*, May 2019, pp. 71–80.

14. Kenneth J. Arrow, "Uncertainty and the Welfare Economics of Medical Care," *The American Economic Review* 53, no. 5 (1963): 941–73.

15. Otto, *Teeth*, p. 99.

16. "Dossier on Periodontal Disease," European Federation on Periodontology, https://www.efp.org/publications/EFP_Dossier_on_Periodontal_Disease_2018.pdf.

17. "Cochrane US," Cochrane, https://us.cochrane.org.

18. "American Pediatric Dentists," American Pediatric Dentists, https://www.aapd.org.

19. "Dental Care Health Professional Shortage Areas (HPSAs)," Kaiser Family Foundation, last updated December 31, 2018, https://www.kff.org/other/state-indicator/dental-care-health-professional-shortage-areas-hpsas/?currentTimeframe=0&sortModel=%7B%22colId%22:%22Location%22,%22sort%22:%22asc%22%7D.

CHAPTER 15

1. "50 Years of Medicare; How Did We Get Here?" The Commonwealth Fund, https://interactives.commonwealthfund.org/medicare-timeline/.

2. "Medicare Timeline," Kaiser Family Foundation, last modified March 24, 2015, https://www.kff.org/medicare/timeline/medicare-timeline/.

3. Juliette Cubanski, Tricia Neuman, and Meredith Freed, "The Facts on Medicare Spending and Financing," Kaiser Family Foundation, last modified August 20, 2019, https://www.kff.org/medicare/issue-brief/the-facts-on-medicare-spending-and-financing/.

4. Ibid.

5. Ibid.

6. "Medicare Enrollment Dashboard," Centers for Medicare & Medicaid Services, https://www.cms.gov/Research-Statistics-Data-and-Systems/Statistics-Trends-and-Reports/Dashboard/Medicare-Enrollment/Enrollment%20Dashboard.html.

7. Gretchen Jacobson, Meredith Freed, Anthony Damico, and Tricia Neuman, "A Dozen Facts about Medicare Advantage in 2019," Kaiser Family Foundation, last modified June 6, 2019, www.kff.org/medicare/issue-brief/a-dozen-facts-about-medicare-advantage-in-2019.

8. Ibid.

9. "2019 Medicare Advantage and Part D Prescription Drug Program Landscape," Fact Sheet, Centers for Medicare & Medicaid Services, September 28, 2019, https://www.cms.gov/newsroom/fact-sheets/2019-medicare-advantage-and-part-d-prescription-drug-program-landscape.

10. "Medicare," Kaiser Family Foundation, www.kff.org/state-category/medicare/.

11. "An Overview of Medicare," Kaiser Family Foundation, February 13, 2019, https://www.kff.org/medicare/issue-brief/an-overview-of-medicare/.

12. Hillary Hoffower, "Medicare Isn't Enough for Retirees—Here's How Much Extra Coverage Costs in Every State, Ranked," *Business Insider,* June 17, 2018, https://www.businessinsider.com/how-much-medigap-plans-cost-every-state-ranked-2018-6.

13. Cubanski, Neuman, and Freed, "The Facts on Medicare Spending and Financing."

14. Rachel Fehr, Cynthia Cox, and Larry Levitt, "Insurer Participation on ACA Marketplaces, 2014–2019," Kaiser Family Foundation, November 14, 2018, https://www.kff.org/health-reform/issue-brief/insurer-participation-on-aca-marketplaces-2014-2019/.

15. Gretchen Johnson, Anthony Damico, Tricia Neuman, "Medicare Advantage 2019 Spotlight: First Look," Kaiser Family Foundation, October 16, 2018, https://www.kff.org/report-section/medicare-advantage-2019-spotlight-first-look-data-note/.

16. "2019 Medicare Advantage and Part D Prescription Drug Program Landscape."

17. Ibid.

18. Shanoor Seervai, "Cuts to the ACA's Outreach Budget Will Make It Harder for People to Enroll," The Commonwealth Fund, October 11, 2017, https://www.commonwealthfund.org/publications/other-publication/2017/oct/cuts-acas-outreach-budget-will-make-it-harder-people-enroll?redirect_source=/publications/publication/2017/oct/cuts-acas-outreach-budget-will-make-it-harder-people-enroll.

19. "Medicare and You," Center for Medicare and Medicaid Services, 2019, https://www.medicare.gov/sites/default/files/2018-09/10050-medicare-and-you.pdf.

20. "Local Medicare Help," State Health Insurance Assistance Programs, https://www.shiptacenter.org.

21. "State Health Insurance Assistance Program," Congressional Research Services, February 4, 2019, https://crsreports.congress.gov/product/pdf/IF/IF10623.

22. "Grants Awarded for the Federally-Facilitated Exchange Navigator Program," Press Release, CMS.gov, September 12, 2018, https://www.cms.gov/newsroom/press-releases/grants-awarded-federally-facilitated-exchange-navigator-program.

23. Jacobson, Freed, Damico, and Neuman, "A Dozen Facts about Medicare Advantage in 2019."

24. Ibid.

25. Cubanski, Neuman, and Freed, "The Facts on Medicare Spending and Financing."

26. Dan Diamond, "Medicare's Cost Surprise: It's Going Down," *Politico*, September 12, 2018, https://www.politico.com/agenda/story/2018/09/12/medicare-spending-cost-budget-000692.

27. "Who Is Eligible for Medicare?" HHS.gov, September 11, 2014, https://www.hhs.gov/answers/medicare-and-medicaid/who-is-elibible-for-medicare/index.html.

28. Edward Berchick, "Who Are the Uninsured?" *Census Blogs*, September 14, 2017, https://www.census.gov/newsroom/blogs/random-samplings/2017/09/who_are_the_uninsure.html.

29. Justin McCarthy, "Most Americans Still Rate Their Healthcare Quite Positively," Gallup, December 7, 2018, https://news.gallup.com/poll/245195/americans-rate-healthcare-quite-positively.aspx.

30. "An Overview of Medicare."

31. Juliette Cubanski, Wyatt Koma, Anthony Damico, and Tricia Neuman, "How Many Seniors Live in Poverty?" Kaiser Family Foundation, November 19, 2018, https://www.kff.org/medicare/issue-brief/how-many-seniors-live-in-poverty/.

32. Ibid.

33. Robin Osborn, Michelle M Doty, Donald Moulds, Dana O. Sarnak, and Arnav Shah, "Older Americans Were Sicker and Faced More Financial Barriers to Health Care Than Counterparts in Other Countries," *Health Affairs* 36, no. 12 (2017): 2123–32.

34. Tatjiana Meschede, Lauren Bercaw, Laura Sullivan, and Martha Cronin, "Post-Recession Senior Insecurity Remains High," Living Longer on Less Series, Institute on Assets and Social Policy, The Heller School on Social Policy and Management, Brandeis University, February 2015, https://heller.brandeis.edu/iasp/pdfs/racial-wealth-equity/loll/post-reces sion-senior-insecurity.pdf.

35. Jeffrey M. Jones, "Healthcare Costs Top Financial Problem for U.S. Families," Gallup, May 30, 2019, https://news.gallup.com/poll/257906/ healthcare-costs-top-financial-problem-families.aspx.

36. Lance Stevens and Lawrence Mallory, "U.S. Seniors Pay Bill, Yet Many Cannot Afford Healthcare," Gallup Blog, April 15, 2019, https:// news.gallup.com/opinion/gallup/248741/seniors-pay-billions-yet-cannot- afford-healthcare.aspx.

37. G. Marshall, S. Lewis, S. Szanton, K. L. Stansbury, and R. Thorpe, "Financial Hardship and Psychological Distress among Middle Aged and Older Americans," *The Gerontologist* 55, Suppl. 2 (2015): 428.

38. Meredith Freed, Tricia Neuman, and Gretchen Jacobson, "Drilling Down on Dental Coverage and Costs for Medicare Beneficiaries," Kaiser Family Foundation, March 13, 2019, https://www.kff.org/medicare/issue- brief/drilling-down-on-dental-coverage-and-costs-for-medicare-benefi ciaries/.

39. Krishna Aravamudhan, Melissa Burroughs, Jeffrey Chaffin, Elisa M. Chávez, Jennifer Goldberg, Judith Jones, Kata Kertesz, Wey-Wey Kwok, Richard Manski, Michael Monopoli, Cheryl Fish-Parcham, David Preble, Bianca Rogers, Beth Truett, Marko Vujicic, Patrick Willard, and Cassan- dra Yarbrough, "An Oral Health Benefit in Medicare Part B: It's Time to Include Oral Health in Health Care," Oral Health America, 2018, https:// familiesusa.org/sites/default/files/product_documents/Medicare_Dental_ White_Paper.pdf.

40. Freed, Neuman, and Jacobson, "Drilling Down on Dental Coverage."

41. "Older Americans Need Better Access to Dental Care," Fact Sheet, The Pew Charitable Trusts, July 2016, https://www.pewtrusts.org/-/media/ assets/2016/07/olderamericans_fs_final.pdf.

42. Ibid.

43. Michael S. Finke, John S. Howe, and Sandra J. Huston, "Old Age and the Decline in Financial Literacy," *Management Science* 63, no. 1 (2017): 213–30.

44. W. Bruine De Bruin, A. Parker, and B. Fischhoff, "Explaining Adult Age Differences in Decision-Making Competence," *Journal of Behavioral Decision Making* 25, no. 4 (2012): 352–60.

45. David I. Laibson, Sumit Agarwal, John C. Driscoll, and Xavier Gabaix, "The Age of Reason: Financial Decisions over the Life-Cycle with Implications for Regulation," *Brookings Papers on Economic Activity*, no. 2 (2009): 51–117.

46. J. H. Hibbard, P. Slovic, E. Peters, M. L. Finucane, and M. Tusler, "Is the Informed-Choice Policy Approach Appropriate for Medicare Beneficiaries?" *Health Affairs* 20, no. 3 (2001): 199–203.

47. "Medicare Timeline."

48. "One-Fourth of Adults and Nearly Half of Adults under 30 Don't Have a Primary Care Doctor," Kaiser Family Foundation, February 8, 2019, https://www.kff.org/other/slide/one-fourth-of-adults-and-nearly-half-of-adults-under-30-dont-have-a-primary-care-doctor/.

49. Sandra G. Boodman, "Spurred by Convenience, Millennials Often Spurn the 'Family Doctor' Model," *Kaiser Health News*, October 9, 2018, https://khn.org/news/spurred-by-convenience-millennials-often-spurn-the-family-doctor-model/.

50. 2019 AAFP/CompHealth Physician Happiness Survey, American Academy of Family Physicians and CompHealth, March 19, 2019, https://comphealth.com/resources/physician-happiness-survey/.

51. Jeff Stein, "Does Bernie Sanders's Health Plan Cost $33 Trillion—or Save $2 Trillion?" *Washington Post*, July 31, 2018, https://www.washingtonpost.com/business/economy/does-bernie-sanderss-health-plan-cost-33-trillion--or-save-2-trillion/2018/07/31/d178b14e-9432-11e8-a679-b09212fb69c2_story.html.

CHAPTER 16

1. Adora Svitak, "What Wisdom Can Adults Learn from Kids?" Interview by Guy Raz, TED Radio Hour, National Public Radio, June 10, 2016, https://www.npr.org/templates/transcript/transcript.php?storyId=481293037.

2. Adora Svitak, "What Adults Can Learn from Kids," Filmed February 13, 2010, in Palm Springs, CA, TED video, 8:12. https://www.ted.com/talks/adora_svitak/ transcript.

Index

About the Author

Deborah Dove Gordon is a seasoned health care executive and former chief marketing officer of a nationally ranked health plan. She is a fellow in the fifth class of the Aspen Institute's Health Innovators Fellowship, an Eisenhower fellow, and a former senior fellow at the Harvard Kennedy School. She earned a BA in bioethics at Brown University and an MBA with distinction at the Harvard Business School.